BLUEPRINTS
Orthopedics

Blueprints **for your pocket!**

In an effort to answer the need for high-yield review books for elective rotations, Blackwell Publishing now brings you Blueprints in pocket size.

These new Blueprints provide the essential content needed during the shorter rotations. They also provide the basic content needed for USMLE Steps 2 and 3, or if you were unable to fit in the rotation, these new pocket-sized Blueprints are just what you need.

Each book focuses on the high-yield essential content for the most commonly encountered problems of the specialty. Each book features these special appendices:

- Career and residency opportunities
- Commonly prescribed medications
- Self-test Q&A section

Ask for these at your medical bookstore or check them out online at www.blackwellmedstudent.com

Blueprints Anasthesiology
Blueprints Dermatology
Blueprints Infectious Diseases
Blueprints Gastroenterology
Blueprints Hematology and Oncology
Blueprints Ophthalmology
Blueprints Orthopedics
Blueprints Pediatric ICU
Blueprints Pediatric Infectious Diseases
Blueprints Plastic Surgery
Blueprints Urology

BLUEPRINTS
Orthopedics

Grant Cooper, MD
Resident, Department of Physical Medicine and Rehabilitation
New York-Presbyterian Hospital
The University Hospitals of Columbia and Cornell
New York, New York

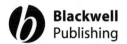
Blackwell
Publishing

Blackwell Publishing, Inc., 350 Main Street,
Malden, Massachusetts 02148-5018, USA
Blackwell Publishing Ltd, 9600 Garsington Road, Oxford OX4 2DQ, UK
Blackwell Publishing Asia Pty Ltd, 550 Swanston Street,
Carlton, Victoria 3053, Australia

05 06 07 08 5 4 3 2 1

ISBN-13: 978-1-4051-0401-2
ISBN-10: 1-4051-0401-5

Library of Congress Cataloging-in-Publication Data

Cooper, Grant, M.D.
  Blueprints orthopedics/Grant Cooper
    p. ; cm.—(Blueprints)
  Includes index.
  ISBN-10: 1-4051-0401-5 (pbk. : alk. paper)
  ISBN-13: 978-1-4051-0401-2 (pbk. : alk. paper)   1. Orthopedics—
Outlines, syllabi, etc.
  [DNLM: 1. Orthopedic Procedures—Handbooks. WE 39 C776b 2005]
I. Title.   II. Series.
RD732.7.C66 2005
161.7'0076—dc22   2005006972

A catalogue record for this title is available from the British Library

Acquisitions: Beverly Copland
Development: Kate Heinle
Production: Debra Murphy
Cover design: Hannus Design Associates
Interior design: Mary McKeon
Typesetter: International Typesetting and Composition in Ft. Lauderdale, FL
Printed and bound by Capital City Press in Berlin, VT

For further information on Blackwell Publishing, visit our website:
www.blackwellmedstudent.com

Notice: The indications and dosages of all drugs in this book have been recommended in the medical literature and conform to the practices of the general community. The medications described do not necessarily have specific
approval by the Food and Drug Administration for use in the diseases and
dosages for which they are recommended. The package insert for each drug
should be consulted for use and dosage as approved by the FDA. Because
standards for usage change, it is advisable to keep abreast of revised recommendations, particularly those concerning new drugs.

The publisher's policy is to use permanent paper from mills that operate a
sustainable forestry policy, and which has been manufactured from pulp
processed using acid-free and elementary chlorine-free practices.
Furthermore, the publisher ensures that the text paper and cover board
used have met acceptable environmental accreditation standards.

To Jason, Sharon, Reuven, Aaron, Alan, Suzanne, Allan, Carol, Robin, John, Emma, Allison, Dragomir, Ljubica, and Viktor, for always being there and supporting me.

To my parents, for leading by example, and for teaching me to strive to do the same.

To Ana, for giving it meaning.

Contents

Reviewers ....*x*
Preface ....*xi*
Note to the Reader ....*xii*
Acknowledgments ....*xiii*
Abbreviations ....*xiv*
Normal Laboratory Values ....*xvi*

Chapter 1: Cervical Spine 1
  High-Yield Surgical and Functional Anatomy 1
  Cervical Radiculopathy 3
  Cervical Spondylotic Myelopathy 6
  Axial Neck Pain and Cervical Zygapophyseal (Z)
  Joint Disease 7
  Spondylolisthesis of the Axis 8
  Atlanto-Occipital Dislocation 9
  Atlas Fracture 10
  Atlantoaxial Rotary Subluxation 11
  Odontoid Fracture 11

Chapter 2: Shoulder 13
  High-Yield Surgical and Functional Anatomy 13
  Shoulder Instability 15
  Adhesive Capsulitis 18
  Impingement Syndrome and Rotator Cuff Disease 19
  Long Head of the Biceps Disorders 23
  Rotator Cuff Calcific Tendonitis 25
  Acromioclavicular Joint Injuries 26
  Clavicular Fracture 27
  Humeral Shaft Fracture 28

Chapter 3: Elbow and Forearm 30
  High-Yield Surgical and Functional Anatomy 30
  Lateral and Medial Epicondylitis 31
  Ulnar Collateral Ligament Injury 33
  Osteochondritis Dissecans 34

Cubital Tunnel Syndrome 35
Distal Humeral Shaft Fracture 36
Supracondylar Fracture 37
Radial Head Fracture 39
Monteggia Fracture 40

Chapter 4: Wrist and Hand **42**
High-Yield Surgical and Functional Anatomy 42
Carpal Tunnel Syndrome 43
De Quervain's Tenosynovitis 46
Stenosing Tenosynovitis 48
Rheumatoid Arthritis 49
Ganglion 50
Kienbock's Disease 52
Distal Radius Fracture 52
Scaphoid Fracture 53

Chapter 5: Thoracolumbar Spine **56**
High-Yield Surgical and Functional Anatomy 56
Adolescent Idiopathic Scoliosis 57
Low Back Pain 58
Lumbosacral Radiculopathy 62
Dysplastic and Isthmic Spondylolisthesis 68
Osteoporotic Vertebral Compression Fracture 70

Chapter 6: Hip **73**
High-Yield Surgical and Functional Anatomy 73
Developmental Dysplasia of the Hip 74
Legg-Calvé-Perthes Disease 77
Transient Synovitis 79
Slipped Capital Femoral Epiphysis 81
Osteoarthritis of the Hip 83
Rheumatoid Arthritis of the Hip 86
Hip Dislocation 87
Hip Fracture 89

Chapter 7: Knee **94**
High-Yield Surgical and Functional Anatomy 94
Osgood-Schlatter Disease 95
Osteochondritis Dissecans 96
Anterior Cruciate Ligament Injury 97
Medial Collateral Ligament Injury 99

Posterior Cruciate Ligament Injury 101
Meniscus Injuries 102
Knee Osteoarthritis 105
Patellofemoral Disorders 108
Patella Fracture 110
Tibial Plateau Fracture 111

Chapter 8: Ankle and Foot 113
High-Yield Surgical and Functional Anatomy 113
Equinovarus Deformity 114
Ankle Sprain 114
Achilles Tendon Injuries 117
Osteochondritis Dissecans 118
Anterior Bony Impingement 119
Plantar Fasciitis 120
Hallux Valgus 121
Hallux Rigidus 122
Interdigital Neuroma 123
Distal Tibial Fracture 123
Calcaneal Fracture 127
Talus Fracture 127

Appendix A: Opportunities in Orthopedics *130*
Appendix B: Review Questions and Answers *132*
Appendix C: Commonly Prescribed Medications
(Adult Doses) *153*
Appendix D: Glossary of Key Words, Terms, and Tests *155*
Appendix E: Suggested Additional Reading *159*
Index *164*

Reviewers

Simon Chao, MD
Resident, Orthopaedic Surgery
Temple University Hospital
Philadelphia, Pennsylvania

Alexis Dang, MD
Resident, Orthopaedic Surgery
University of California, San Francisco
San Francisco, California

Michael W. Kessler
Class of 2005
Albany Medical College
Albany, New York

Christopher McAndrew, MD
Resident, Orthopaedic Surgery
University Hospitals of Cleveland/
    Case Western Reserve University
Cleveland, Ohio

B.K. Parsley, MD
Resident, Division of Orthopaedics
Southern Illinois University
Springfield, Illinois

Esben Vogelius
Class of 2006
University of Medicine and Dentistry of New Jersey/
    New Jersey Medical School
Highland Park, New Jersey

Preface

Blueprints have become the standard for medical students to use during their clerkship rotations and subinternships and as review books for taking the USMLE Steps 2 and 3.

Blueprints initially were only available for the five main specialties: medicine, pediatrics, obstetrics and gynecology, surgery, and psychiatry. Students found these books so valuable that they asked for Blueprints in other topics and so family medicine, emergency medicine, neurology, cardiology, and radiology were added.

In an effort to answer a need for high-yield review books for the elective rotations, Blackwell Publishing now brings you Blueprints in pocket size. These books are developed to provide students in the shorter, elective rotations, often taken in 4th year, with the same high-yield, essential contents of the larger Blueprint books. These new pocket-sized Blueprints will be invaluable for those students who need to know the essentials of a clinical area but were unable to take the rotation. Students in physician assistant, nurse practitioner, and osteopath programs will find these books meet their needs for the clinical specialties.

Feedback from student reviewers gives high praise for this addition to the Blueprint brand. Each of these new books was developed to be read in a short time period and to address the basics needed during a particular clinical rotation. Please see the Series Page for a list of the books that will soon be in your bookstore.

Note to the Reader

The purpose of this book is to provide you with a high-yield review of the most important concepts and topics in orthopedics. Ideally, this book could be read and reread in the weeks or week (or even weekend) before your orthopedic rotation. If you are about to embark on your first orthopedic rotation, this book will offer you an introduction to the important topics that you will need to know during your rotation. If you have already done one or more orthopedic rotations, reading this book will help you recall the highest yield points of orthopedics and keep them fresh in your mind. For all students and residents, this book could be easily stored in the pocket of your white coat and used as a means of quick reference and review of pertinent topics before seeing your patients, rounding with your team, or going into the operating room. This book is not intended as a comprehensive review of orthopedics. This book is an overall introduction to the highest yield points, and is intended to provide you with a good quick review. However, as you learn more and progress in your training, you should supplement this text with other texts and resources for a more thorough and detailed understanding of orthopedics.

A note on chapter organization: Orthopedic texts are organized in a variety of ways. Although many orthopedic texts are organized with different chapters for pediatrics, trauma, emergencies, and other specific subcategories of disorders, the organization of this book has been kept strictly anatomic. For example, when you have a patient with slipped capital femoral epiphysis (SCFE), you do not need to wonder if the disorder is to be found in the hip section, pediatric section, or emergency section—it will be in the hip section. The decision to keep the organization of this book anatomic was done in order to offer you the quickest and easiest referencing source possible.

Acknowledgments

There are many people who made this book possible. To Beverly Copland and Kate Heinle, my two superb editors, thank you for your valuable feedback, enthusiasm, vision, and unwavering support for this book. Thank you also to the reviewers for their important feedback.

—Grant Cooper, MD

Abbreviations

ACDF	Anterior cervical discectomy and fusion
ACI	Autologous chondrocyte implantation
AC joint	Acromioclavicular joint
ACL	Anterior cruciate ligament
ANA	Antinuclear antibody
AP	Anteroposterior
APTT	Activated partial thromboplastin time
ATFL	Anterior talofibular ligament
AVN	Avascular necrosis
BUN	Blood urea nitrogen
CBC	Complete blood count
CFL	Calcaneofibular ligament
CLBP	Chronic low back pain
CPM	Continuous passive motion
CTLSO	Cervicothoracolumbosacral orthosis
CT scan	Computed tomography scan
DDH	Developmental dysplasia of the hip
DIP	Distal interphalangeal
DVT	Deep venous thrombosis
ESR	Erythrocyte sedimentation rate
Hct	Hematocrit
Hgb	Hemoglobin
IDET	Intradiscal electrothermal annuloplasty
INR	International Normalized Ratio
LBP	Low back pain
LCPD	Legg-Calvé-Perthes disease
MCL	Medial collateral ligament
MRI	Magnetic resonance imaging
NSAIDs	Nonsteroidal anti-inflammatory drugs
OA	Osteoarthritis
OCD	Osteochondritis dissecans
ORIF	Open reduction internal fixation
PA	Posteroanterior
PCL	Posterior cruciate ligament
PE	Pulmonary embolus
PIP	Proximal interphalangeal
PMMA	Polymethylmethacrylate
PT	Prothrombin time

PTFL	Posterior talofibular ligament
PTT	Partial thromboplastin time
Q-angle	Quadriceps angle
RA	Rheumatoid arthritis
RF	Rheumatoid factor
SCFE	Slipped capital femoral epiphysis
SLAP	Superior labral anterior posterior
THR	Total hip replacement
TKR	Total knee replacement
TLSO	Thoracolumbosacral orthosis
TS	Transient synovitis
URI	Upper respiratory tract infection
US	Ultrasonography
WBC	White blood cell count
Z-joint	Zygapophyseal joint

Normal Laboratory Values

Activated partial thromboplastin time (APTT): 25–39 seconds
Albumin: 3.2–5.0 g/dl
Blood urea nitrogen (BUN): 7–25
Creatinine: 0.7–1.4
Hematocrit (Hct) in adult female: 37–41%
Hematocrit (Hct) in adult male: 40–54%
Hemoglobin (Hgb) in adult female: 12–16 g/dl
Hemoglobin (Hgb) in adult male: 14–18 g/dl
International normalized ratio (INR): 1.0–1.4
International normalized ratio (INR) (therapeutic): 2–3
Partial thromboplastin time (PTT): 30–45 seconds
Platelet count: 130–400 thousand/mcl
Prothrombin time (PT): 10–13 seconds
White blood cell (WBC): 3.8–11 thousand/mcl

Cervical Spine

High-Yield Surgical and Functional Anatomy

The cervical spine serves three important functions: (1) to support and stabilize the head, (2) to provide range of motion to the head, and (3) to safely house the spinal cord and vertebral artery. There are seven cervical vertebrae. The atlanto-occipital joint articulates the skull and C1 vertebra (also called the *atlas*). The atlantoaxial joint articulates between C1 and C2 (also called the *axis*). The cervical zygapophyseal (Z) joints are paired synovial joints articulating between the inferior articular processes of one joint with the superior articular processes of the adjacent inferior vertebra. The anterior longitudinal ligament is a strong, fibrous band connecting the anterior aspects of the vertebral bodies and intervertebral discs. The cervical spine is classically reached via either an anterior or posterior surgical approach.

■ Anterior Approach

The anterior approach to the cervical vertebrae is used for excision of herniated discs, fusion surgery, drainage of abscesses, and other pathologies. Superficial structures that may be palpated for convenient landmarks include the hyoid bone, palpated at the level of C3; the thyroid cartilage, palpated at the level of C4 and C5; and the cricoid cartilage, palpated at the level of C6. The sternocleidomastoid muscle is a broad, superficial muscle that is also easily palpated. The sternocleidomastoid muscle arises from the manubrium of the sternum and medial third of the clavicle, and it attaches to the lateral part of the mastoid process and occipital bone. The sternocleidomastoid is innervated by the spinal accessory nerve (cranial nerve XI) and second and third cervical nerves. The sternocleidomastoid laterally flexes the neck when acting unilaterally and, when acting bilaterally flexes the neck. A convenient way to test the sternocleidomastoid muscle is to have the patient flex the head against resistance.

The platysma muscle is another important superficial muscle in the anterior neck. The platysma is a thin muscle that arises from the overlying fascia and skin on the pectoralis major and deltoid muscles. It inserts into the inferior mandible and lower face.

The platysma is innervated by the facial nerve (cranial nerve VII). The platysma tenses the skin and draws the corner of the mouth in an inferior direction. The platysma is a critical muscle for facial expression, and its injury (or the injury of its nerve supply) during surgery can result in facial deformity.

The carotid sheath is a tubular fascial fusion of the fascial extensions of the cervical and prevertebral fascia. It encloses the vagus nerve (cranial nerve X) posteriorly, common carotid artery medially, and internal jugular vein laterally. In addition, deep cervical lymph nodes are found. The cervical portion of the sympathetic trunk is found posterior to the carotid sheath. The recurrent laryngeal nerve is a branch of the vagus nerve and is protected by the longus colli muscle.

The anterior longitudinal ligament is a white structure that extends from the atlas (C1) inferiorly to the pelvic surface. The anterior longitudinal ligament is larger than the posterior longitudinal ligament and connects the anterior portions of the intervertebral discs and vertebral bodies. An important structural responsibility of the anterior longitudinal ligament is to prevent cervical hyperextension.

■ Posterior Approach

The posterior surgical approach to the cervical spine is used for fusion surgery, excision of herniated discs, nerve root exploration, and other pathologies. The spinous processes are easily palpated superficial structures. C7 is the largest spinous process. To differentiate C7 from T1, laterally rotate the patient's head. C7 will move slightly, but T1 is fixed and will not move. As the dissection begins, the paraspinal cervical muscles are identified. The paraspinal cervical muscles are concerned primarily with posture, movement, and support of the neck and head. The trapezius muscle constitutes the superficial layer. The trapezius is a large, triangular muscle. It arises from the occipital bone, ligamentum nuchae, and the spines of the seventh cervical vertebrae and all the thoracic vertebrae. It attaches to the lateral third of the clavicle, acromion, and spine of the scapula. The trapezius is innervated by the spinal part of the accessory nerve (cranial nerve XI). The trapezius can pull the scapula superior, medial, and inferior, with its upper, middle, and lower fibers, respectively. A convenient way to test the trapezius is to instruct the patient to lift the shoulders up against resistance.

The splenius muscles are deep to the trapezius and arise from the inferior half of the ligamentum nuchae and the spinous processes of T1-T6 vertebrae, and they insert into the mastoid process, occipital bone, and C1-C4. The splenius muscles serve to laterally flex and/or extend the head. The splenius muscles are innervated by the dorsal rami of the inferior cervical nerves. A convenient way to test these muscles is to have the patient laterally flex the head against resistance.

Deep to the cervical muscles and the spinous processes is the ligamentum flavum. The ligamentum flavum connects the adjacent cervical laminae. The zygapophyseal joints, formed by the adjacent inferior and superior articular processes, are innervated by the medial branches of the dorsal rami. The blue-white matter deep to the ligamentum flavum is the dura. Within the vertebral canal, the posterior longitudinal ligament attaches the intervertebral discs and the posterior vertebral bodies from the axis (C2) superiorly extending inferiorly to the sacrum.

Cervical Radiculopathy

A radiculopathy is caused by compression of the nerve root. Nerve roots may be compressed by several pathologies, including foraminal stenosis from disc herniation (most common cause), an osteophyte on the zygapophyseal joint, or vertical subluxation of the vertebrae. When considering cervical radiculopathy, it is important to remember that the cervical nerve roots 1 to 7 exit above their corresponding numbered pedicles. So, for example, the C4 nerve root exits between the C3 and C4 vertebrae. C8, however, exits between C7 and T1, and T1 exits between T1 and T2. Therefore, a C3-4 disc herniation will typically result in a C4 radiculopathy. Likewise, a T1-2 disc herniation (relatively uncommon) will result in a T1 radiculopathy. Radiculopathies are often (though not always) associated with radicular pain. Radicular pain is caused by inflammation of a nerve root or compression of the dorsal root ganglion.

■ Clinical Manifestations

The typical patient presents with a complaint of shooting electric pain, numbness, tingling, burning, weakness, and/or dysesthesia in the shoulder and/or arm. The distribution of symptoms depends on the nerve root level of compression (Table 1-1).

Physical Examination

Sensory testing should be performed in all patients. Patients may report numbness over the involved areas of distribution for the involved particular nerve root (Figure 1-1). Spurling's test is typically performed during the evaluation of a radiculopathy. In this test, the neck is extended and rotated to the side of suspected pathology. Gentle axial compression is applied (Figure 1-2). This maneuver narrows the foramen and should reproduce symptoms in a patient with a true radiculopathy. When symptoms are

■ TABLE 1-1 Distribution of Sensory, Muscle, and Reflex Involvement for Different Neurologic Levels

Neurologic Level	Sensory Distribution	Weakness	Reflex Involved
C2 or C3	Subocciput region of the head	None	None
C4	Trapezius	Trapezius	
C5	Lateral shoulder, lateral elbow crease	Shoulder abduction and elbow flexion	Biceps
C6	Lateral forearm, first and second digits	Elbow flexion and wrist extension	Brachioradialis
C7	Arm and third digit	Wrist flexion and elbow extension	Triceps
C8	Four and fifth digits	Finger flexion	None
T1	Medial elbow crease	Finger abduction ("clumsiness" due to intrinsic hand muscles)	None

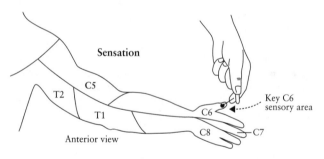

Figure 1-1 • Dermatomal distribution (anterior view) of sensory testing. (Reproduced with permission from Gross, J. *Musculoskeletal Examination,* second edition. Figure 4.62, p. 74. Blackwell Publishing, 2002).

reproduced, the patient is said to have a positive Spurling's test. Reciprocally, relieving the pressure from the foramen should alleviate symptoms. This is accomplished with gentle traction and rotation of the neck to the opposite side with the neck placed in flexion. Muscle and reflex testing should also be performed and will reveal weakness and sluggish reflexes in the involved areas of distribution (see Table 1-1).

All patients should also be evaluated for long tract signs (Hoffman's, Babinski's) to rule out more serious pathology.

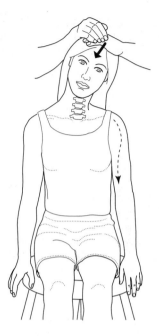

Figure 1-2 • The Spurling test being performed. (Reproduced with permission from Gross, J. *Musculoskeletal Examination*, second edition. Figure 4.67, p. 78. Blackwell Publishing, 2002).

■ Diagnostic Evaluation

Plain films with anteroposterior (AP) and lateral views should be taken in flexion and extension. If anterior displacement of the pharyngeal air shadow is noted, there is likely soft tissue swelling and possible disruption of the intervertebral disc or anterior longitudinal ligament. However, to fully define the anatomy and pathology, magnetic resonance imaging (MRI) needs to be obtained. Electrodiagnostic studies may also be helpful in the final analysis to delineate the precise nerve involvement.

■ Treatment

The mainstay of treatment for cervical radiculopathy is conservative. Initial conservative care includes nonsteroidal anti-inflammatory drugs (NSAIDs), physical therapy including stretching and strengthening exercises, and epidural steroid injections. Epidural steroid injections are administered under fluoroscopic guidance using either an interlaminar or transforaminal approach.

Patients with severe, persistent symptoms or patients with progressive neurologic deficits merit surgical consideration. A typical surgical approach is an anterior cervical discectomy and fusion (ACDF). Using this approach, the intervertebral disc is dissected. If a fragment of the disc has protruded posterior to the posterior longitudinal ligament, it may be necessary to resect the posterior longitudinal ligament as well. Posterior approaches are less common but are sometimes used for bilateral radiculopathy or radiculopathy at more than one level.

Cervical Spondylotic Myelopathy

Cervical spondylotic myelopathy is created by a spinal cord impingement. The impingement of the spinal cord may be from bony overgrowth, disc, or other tissue. It typically occurs in patients who already have a congenitally narrowed canal. In contrast to radiculopathy, cervical myelopathy does not have a good prognosis with conservative management.

■ Clinical Manifestations

The typical patient complains of axial neck pain and radicular symptoms. Symptoms are typically consistent with an anterior cord syndrome. In this syndrome, there are more motor deficits in the lower extremities. The typical patient will therefore have problems with balance and weakness in the lower extremities. Weakness may or may not be present in the upper extremities. Fine motor function such as grasping may be impaired in some patients, leading them to complain of "clumsy hands."

In other patients, however, symptoms may be consistent with a central cord syndrome. In this syndrome, motor deficits are greater in the upper extremity. When bowel or bladder function is disturbed, it is a reflection of significant disease progression and an indicator of a poor prognosis.

Physical Examination
On examination, the patient may have a wide-based and/or unsteady gait. The patient may have a positive *Lhermitte's sign*, in which flexing the neck produces an electric shock sensation down the arms and legs. The patient may also have *dysdiadochokinesis* (the inability to perform rapid, alternating movements). The patient may have hyper-reflexive reflexes. The long tract signs of Babinski and Hoffman may be positive.

To elicit Hoffman's sign, stabilize the patient's third digit's proximal interphalangeal (PIP) joint and briskly flick the distal phalanx. A positive Hoffman's sign occurs if the interphalangeal joint of the thumb or the distal interphalangeal (DIP) joint of the second digit reflexively flexes.

To elicit Babinski's sign, a sharp instrument is run across the plantar surface of the patient's foot. The instrument traces the lateral border of the foot from the calcaneus to the first digit. If the first toe reflexively extends and the rest of the toes flex, the test is considered positive and the patient has a Babinski reflex. In patients without a lesion, the Babinski reflex disappears around the age of 1 year.

■ Diagnostic Evaluation

Plain film radiographs, computed tomography (CT) scan, and MRI should be obtained. When signal changes are observed in the MRI, the prognosis is poor.

■ Treatment

Surgery is typically indicated. Surgical options include ACDF or corpectomy with strut grafting. Laminoplasty may be performed through a posterior incision if desired.

Axial Neck Pain and Cervical Zygapophyseal (Z) Joint Disease

The most common cause of chronic neck pain is cervical zygapophyseal (Z) joint disease, accounting for approximately 40% of all patients with axial neck pain lasting longer than 3 months. In patients who also report a history of a high-speed motor vehicle accident, the prevalence of cervical Z-joint disease jumps to approximately 80%.

The cervical Z-joints are paired synovial facet joints between the consecutive vertebrae. The most common mechanism of injury of the cervical Z-joints is a motor vehicle accident. Cadaveric experiments have demonstrated that upon impact the lower cervical spine is forced anteriorly and superiorly. After that, the cervical spine is progressively extended until the head is thrown backward into extension. This movement provides substantial compressive and torsion forces on the cervical spine.

■ Clinical Manifestations

The typical patient reports a history of neck pain lasting longer than 3 months. Almost all patients will be able to recall a history of neck trauma at some point in their lives. Many patients will report a history of a motor vehicle accident. The typical patient will report axial neck pain and referred, deep, aching pain in the head, trapezius, scapula, and/or arm. However, in some patients, headache is the sole presenting complaint. It is important to remember that whereas radicular pain is sharp and radiating, referred pain is *dull*, *aching*, and perceived deeply. The area of pain in referral pain patterns is also poorly defined.

Patients should be asked to complete a pain map depicting the distribution of their pain. This map is used to suggest which Z-joint is most likely to be diseased.

Physical Examination

Despite conventional thinking, in general, the physical examination is not helpful in determining which, if any, Z-joint level is involved in a patient's neck pain. In patients in whom radiculopathy cannot be ruled out, Spurling's test and a full neurologic examination should always be performed. Spurling's test is performed by putting the patient's head into oblique extension with gentle axial compression, increasing the pressure on the intervertebral foramen. The test is positive if the patient experiences radicular symptoms in this position.

■ Diagnostic Evaluation

In considering uncomplicated axial neck pain, plain film radiography, CT, and MRI are not typically indicated. These imaging studies may reveal cervical spondylosis and/or osteoarthritis. However, these findings occur at comparable rates in asymptomatic people as they do in symptomatic people. Therefore, their presence is not diagnostic. Instead, the only way to reliably diagnose cervical Z-joint disease is with controlled diagnostic blocks of the medial branches of the cervical dorsal rami innervating the suspected Z-joints. These blocks are performed under fluoroscopic guidance. The blocks are considered positive when the patient obtains 100% short-lasting relief when a shorter-acting anesthetic agent is used (e.g., lidocaine) and longer-lasting relief when a longer-acting anesthetic agent is used (e.g., bupivacaine).

■ Treatment

Cervical Z-joint disease is treated with a percutaneous radiofrequency neurotomy of the nerves supplying the symptomatic joint. This procedure creates high-energy friction in the needle electrode, which produces heat and destroys the nerves. The axons may regenerate with time. If this occurs and symptoms reappear, the procedure may need to be repeated.

Spondylolisthesis of the Axis

Axis spondylolisthesis is divided into three types (Table 1-2). Note that in type IIa the significant angulation reflects a probable disruption in the posterior longitudinal ligament and C2-3 disc.

■ TABLE 1-2   Different Types of Axis Spondylolisthesis and Treatment

Type	Characteristics	Treatment
I	Less than 3 mm of displacement, no angulation	External immobilization using a cervical collar
II	Greater than 3 mm of displacement and angulation	Traction reduction and halo immobilization
IIa	Significant angulation with no anterolisthesis	Gentle manipulation with extension and neutralization in a halo device, no traction
III	Z-joint dislocation permitting anterolisthesis	Open reduction of the Z-joint dislocation and posterior C2-3 fusion

■ Clinical Manifestations

The typical patient offers a history of neck and/or arm symptoms following a motor vehicle accident or other high-energy trauma in which the neck undergoes a combination of extension and axial compression followed by forceful flexion.

Physical Examination

Examination should be deferred until imaging studies are obtained.

■ Diagnostic Evaluation

Lateral plain film radiographs in extension and flexion and CT should be obtained. Flexion and extension should not be forced to more than the patient can tolerate so as to not create additional injury.

■ Treatment

See Table 1-2. Note that in type IIa, traction is strictly contraindicated because of the ligamentous disruption.

Atlanto-Occipital Dislocation

Dislocation of the atlanto-occipital joint results from a hyperextension, distraction, and/or rotational injury. During the injury, excessive force results in osseoligamentous separation of the skull from the spine. Perhaps partly because the atlanto-occipital joint has a more horizontal orientation in children, they are affected twice as often as are adults. Naturally, this injury has potentially devastating consequences, including brainstem dysfunction, cranial nerve deficits, or death.

■ Clinical Manifestations

The typical patient is a child who has just been involved in a motor vehicle accident. The patient may have symptoms of cranial nerve impairment or be unresponsive.

Physical Examination

A brief exam may be performed, including checking for pupillary response. Of course, airway, breathing, and circulation must always be assessed first. The neck should not be manipulated if atlanto-occipital dislocation is suspected. Instead, radiographs should be obtained.

■ Diagnostic Evaluation

Plain film radiographs including AP, lateral, and odontoid views, CT, and/or MRI should be obtained. Subarachnoid hemorrhage at the craniocervical junction seen on MRI is evidence of atlanto-occipital dislocation.

Radiographic evidence is used to classify the dislocation based on the direction of dislocation. Type I is a pure longitudinal dislocation. Type II is the most common type of dislocation and is an anterior dislocation. Type III is a posterior dislocation.

■ Treatment

Because of the loss of ligament stabilizers, traction is contraindicated in type I dislocations. Types II and III may be treated with gentle reduction using 2- to 5-pound weights. Otherwise, halo immobilization with subsequent posterior occipital-cervical fusion is the treatment of choice. The major complications arise from delayed diagnosis and stabilization. Therefore, a low threshold should be used to order the appropriate imaging studies in suspected cases.

Atlas Fracture

Atlas fractures account for up to 13% of all cervical spine fractures and generally occur in response to an axial compression injury with hyperextension, hyperflexion, or forced lateral bending. Typically, the amount of energy required to produce an atlas fracture also results in other fractures. However, when an isolated atlas fracture occurs, the displacement does not generally compress the spinal cord because it displaces in a centrifugal pattern.

■ Clinical Manifestations

The typical patient has suffered an axial compression injury, such as a brick falling from a tall building onto the patient's head, and the patient complains of pain. Football players or other contact athletes may also suffer compression injuries.

Physical Examination

Examination is deferred and radiographs are obtained.

■ Diagnostic Evaluation

Plain film radiographs, including AP and lateral views, and CT are obtained. The fracture is found to be unstable if the transverse atlantal ligament has lost its integrity as measured on lateral films. A greater than 3.5-mm atlanto-dens interval may indicate disruption of the ligament. MRI can be used to better visualize the ligament and directly evaluate for any tears.

■ Treatment

If the fracture is stable, hard collar immobilization may be sufficient. If the fracture is unstable, rigid halo immobilization is used and C1-C2 arthrodesis is often performed.

Atlantoaxial Rotary Subluxation

Atlantoaxial subluxation typically occurs after trauma but may occur spontaneously. Risk factors include a history of rheumatoid arthritis or Down syndrome.

■ Clinical Manifestations

The typical patient presents with a chief complaint of suboccipital pain following an injury and decreased range of motion in the neck.

Physical Examination

On inspection, the patient is seen to hold the head tilted in the direction of the subluxated joint. Radiographs should be obtained before a complete examination.

■ Diagnostic Evaluation

Plain film radiographs and CT should be obtained. The AP film will reveal an asymmetric relationship between the odontoid and the lateral masses of C1. The subluxation is classified based on the imaging findings.

■ Treatment

Refer to Table 1-3 for treatment guidelines.

Odontoid Fracture

Odontoid fractures are associated with a neurologic deficit in up to 25% of cases. The injury usually results from forceful flexion, extension, and/or rotational injury.

■ TABLE 1-3 Atlantoaxial Rotary Subluxation Characteristics and Treatment

Type	Characteristics	Treatment
I	Less than 3 mm of anterior translation, reflecting an intact transverse atlantal ligament	Closed reduction and halo immobilization. If this fails, open reduction
II	3–5 mm of anterior displacement of C1 on C2, reflecting a ruptured transverse atlantal ligament	Atlantoaxial arthrodesis
III	Greater than 5 mm of anterior displacement	Atlantoaxial arthrodesis
IV	Posterior subluxation of C1 on C2	Atlantoaxial arthrodesis

■ Clinical Manifestations

The typical patient reports a history of acute neck pain following significant trauma.

Physical Examination

Exam is deferred until radiographic evaluation.

■ Diagnostic Evaluation

Plain film radiographs and CT imaging are taken and are used to classify the injury. Type I is rare and is an avulsion injury of the alar ligament with oblique fracture at the tip of the dens. Type II is the most common and is a fracture at the base of the dens. Type III is a fracture that extends from the dens all the way to the C2 body.

■ Treatment

Treatment depends on the class of fracture. Type I fractures are externally immobilized for approximately 3 months. After 3 months, repeat imaging studies are obtained in flexion and extension to evaluate for healing. Type II fractures are treated with reduction using traction and halo immobilization. In the elderly, healing is less likely and halo immobilization is less well tolerated. Therefore, elderly patients with type II odontoid fractures are often treated with initial odontoid osteosynthesis. Type III fractures are treated with traction reduction and halo immobilization for 3 months. In the elderly, again, C1-C2 arthrodesis is the initial treatment of choice for many surgeons.

2

Shoulder

High-Yield Surgical and Functional Anatomy

The shoulder is a ball-and-socket synovial joint in which the head of the humerus articulates with the glenoid cavity of the scapula. The shoulder sacrifices stability for mobility, and is in fact the most mobile joint in the body. The deltoid muscle forms the outer muscular layer of the shoulder and, along with the pectoralis major and the latissimus dorsi, provides the power for major shoulder movement. Deep to this layer are the four muscles of the rotator cuff: the supraspinatus, infraspinatus, teres minor, and subscapularis. These muscles may be conveniently remembered by the mnemonic: SITS. The rotator cuff muscles are largely responsible for the stability of the shoulder joint.

■ Anterior Approach

The anterior surgical approach to the shoulder is used for shoulder reconstruction after dislocations, biopsy and excision of tumors, repair of the long head of the biceps tendon, arthroplasty, and other pathologies. Advantages of the anterior approach include excellent joint exposure. Disadvantages include increased bleeding in the skin and subcutaneous tissues.

The deltoid muscle forms the rounded contour of the shoulder. The deltoid has anterior, middle, and posterior fibers that are responsible for shoulder flexion, abduction, and extension, respectively. The deltoid arises from the lateral third of the clavicle, acromion, and the spine of the scapula. It inserts into the deltoid tuberosity in the middle of the lateral portion of the shaft of the humerus. It is innervated by the axillary nerve.

The pectoralis major is another large, superficial muscle. It arises from the medial clavicle, sternum, and first six costal cartilages. It inserts into the lateral lip of the bicipital groove of the humerus. The pectoralis major is innervated by the medial and lateral pectoral nerves. The pectoralis major serves to adduct, flex, and medially rotate the shoulder.

Deep to the pectoralis major and deltoid is the short head of the biceps and coracobrachialis. The coracobrachialis arises from the proximal portion of the coracoid process and inserts into the middle third of the medial surface of the humerus. The biceps brachii arise from the coracoid process and the supraglenoid tubercle of the scapula and insert via the bicipital aponeurosis into the tuberosity of the radius. Both the coracobrachialis and the biceps brachii are innervated by the musculocutaneous nerve. The biceps brachii flexes the elbow and supinates the forearm and both muscles serve to flex the shoulder. The musculocutaneous nerve runs inferior to the coracoid process and is the most superficial nerve of the brachial plexus. Figure 2-1 illustrates the brachial plexus. Injury to the biceps brachii or its nerve supply will result in a lack of elbow flexion.

One of the rotator cuff muscles, the subscapularis muscle, is found deep to the biceps brachii, coracobrachialis, and pectoralis minor. In addition to helping stabilize the shoulder joint, the subscapularis is the rotator cuff muscle responsible for internal rotation. It arises from the subscapular fossa and inserts into the lesser tuberosity of the humerus. It is innervated by the upper and lower subscapular nerves.

If the dissection is performed more lateral, the supraspinatus muscle is found deep to the deltoid. The supraspinatus muscle arises from the supraspinous fossa of the scapula and inserts into

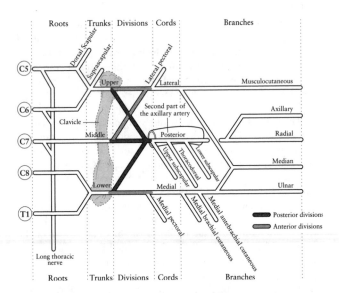

Figure 2-1 • Brachial plexus. (Reproduced with permission from Gross, J. *Musculoskeletal Examination*, second edition. Figure 4.57, p. 69. Blackwell Publishing, 2002).

the greater tuberosity of the humerus. The supraspinatus muscle is responsible for initiation of shoulder abduction. It is innervated by the suprascapular nerve. The tendon of the supraspinatus passes deep to the coracoacromial ligament.

■ Posterior Approach

When dissecting the shoulder from the posterior approach, the infraspinatus and teres minor are found deep to the deltoid. The infraspinatus originates from the infraspinous fossa of the scapula. The teres minor originates from the superolateral border of the scapula. Both muscles insert into the greater tuberosity of the humerus. The teres minor is innervated by the axillary nerve. The infraspinatus is innervated by the suprascapular nerve. Both muscles serve to externally rotate the shoulder. Deep to the infraspinatus and teres minor muscles is the posterior glenoid cavity.

During dissection, if the axillary nerve is injured, the deltoid muscle will be paralyzed, resulting in weakened shoulder abduction, flexion, and extension. In addition, the teres minor will be paralyzed. External rotation of the shoulder will therefore be weakened but, because of the intact infraspinatus, external rotation will not be absent. In addition, there may be a paresthesia over the lateral proximal arm.

Shoulder Instability

Shoulder instability may result from failure of any of the following: the shallow glenoid socket and labrum that holds the humeral head, the glenohumeral ligaments, the coracohumeral ligament, the overhanging coracoacromial arch, and the surrounding and supporting muscles. Approximately 60% to 70% of patients who are younger than 22 years of age who suffer one shoulder dislocation will suffer another. In patients between the ages of 20 and 30, recurrence rates of 50% to 64% have been documented after traumatic anterior instability.

Ninety-five percent of shoulder dislocations dislocate anteriorly. Anterior dislocation typically is caused by an acute injury in which the arm is forced into abduction, external rotation, and extension. This sort of injury often results in a Bankart lesion (a tear of the anterior glenoid labrum) or a Hill-Sachs lesion (compression fracture of the posterior humeral head). Axillary nerve injury also may accompany an anterior shoulder dislocation.

Posterior dislocation is rare and usually results from a violent twisting of the arm in an unusual position (such as that suffered from an electric shock or from a seizure). Patients may also have multidirectional instability.

■ Clinical Manifestations

The typical patient with anterior instability will complain of the shoulder "giving out." The patient may also complain of numbness or weakness during abduction and external rotation. Baseball pitchers may complain of symptom exacerbation during the late cocking phase of pitching during later innings.

A typical patient with posterior instability will complain of pain, numbness, or tingling during arm flexion, adduction, and internal rotation such as happens when pushing open a door.

Physical Examination

A positive apprehension sign is classic of anterior shoulder instability. In this sign, with the patient seated, the examiner puts the patient's arm into abduction, external rotation, and then extension (Figure 2-2). This movement will give the patient the sensation that the humeral head is about to dislocate anteriorly. The patient will react by tensing the body in "apprehension." Repeating the test while applying posteriorly directed pressure to the anterior shoulder (stabilizing the humeral head) alleviates the feeling that the humeral head is slipping out, and the patient's apprehension or tensing of the body is relieved. It is important to complete a full neurovascular evaluation of the patient because shoulder dislocation and relocation may result in neurovascular compromise.

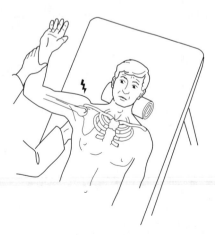

Figure 2-2 • The anterior apprehension test being performed. (Reproduced with permission from Gross, J. *Musculoskeletal Examination,* second edition. Figure 8.89, p. 187. Blackwell Publishing, 2002).

■ Diagnostic Evaluation

Three standard plain radiographic views should be obtained: true anteroposterior (AP), perpendicular to the plane of the scapula, and apical axillary view. An axillary view must be obtained if a posterior dislocation is suspected. The West Point view may be performed to visualize a Bankart lesion. In anterior dislocations, a compression fracture of the posterior humeral head (Hill-Sachs lesion) may be observed on a Stryker's notch view. A Hill-Sachs lesion results from posterior humeral head compression against the anterior glenoid.

Computed tomography (CT) may be obtained to help define potential humeral and glenoid abnormalities. Ultrasound and/or magnetic resonance imaging (MRI) are used to evaluate the rotator cuff for associated injuries in patients older than 40 with weakness or pain found on exam during muscle testing.

■ Differential Diagnosis

• Dislocation
• Subluxation
• Rotator cuff disease

■ Treatment

First-time dislocations are usually treated without surgery. The arm is placed in a sling, radiographs are obtained to confirm adequate reduction, and isometric exercises are begun. Patients may expect to begin a strengthening program in 3 to 4 weeks, with return to preinjury activities at around 3 months. Recurrent anterior instability caused by trauma is treated with activity restriction, bracing, strengthening, and/or surgical intervention. Many physicians advocate for early surgical stabilization in athletes in an effort to minimize the risk of recurrent dislocation and facilitate earlier return to preinjury functional status.

When surgical intervention is used, open procedures are preferred to arthroscopic ones. Arthroscopic repairs carry a higher rate of failure when compared with open procedures. The Bankart procedure with suturing through bone holes is a common and highly effective open procedure that is used for anterior instability repair. In this procedure, rotation is preserved and the labrum is repaired. The most important guiding factors in surgical repair are (1) secure repair of the detached capsule and labrum to the surface of the glenoid, (2) re-creating the fossa-deepening effect of the labrum, and (3) avoidance of excessive tightening of the capsule.

Posterior capsulorrhaphy and posterior glenoid osteotomy are often used for open surgical stabilization of posterior instability.

Multidirectional instability may be surgically treated with the capsular shift. Some surgeons attempt to repair multidirectional instability via an arthroscopic approach with thermal capsular shrinkage and arthroscopic glenoid-based capsular shift with transglenoid suture fixation.

Adhesive Capsulitis

Adhesive capsulitis (frozen shoulder) is a common disorder that, despite much attention, remains relatively poorly understood. The disorder is marked by limitation in passive and active range of motion of the shoulder. On arthroscopy, the synovium of the shoulder has been shown to be inflamed with increased amounts of cytokines, growth factors, and metalloproteinases. These factors are believed to be implicated in the development of adhesive capsulitis.

Risk factors for developing adhesive capsulitis include diabetes mellitus, hypothyroidism, hyperthyroidism, cardiopulmonary disease, cervical disc disease, humeral fractures, biceps tendonitis, rotator cuff disease, and acromioclavicular (AC) disease.

■ Clinical Manifestations

The typical patient is between 40 and 60 years of age and offers a history of a minimal trauma followed by a vague aching in the shoulder and arm. Classically, following the vague aching symptoms, the patient will report the development of a more intense pain that ultimately progresses to difficulty sleeping on the affected arm. After several months, the pain will subside and stiffness will develop on the affected side. If left untreated, the stiffness will progressively worsen over the course of a year as the pain disappears. The stiffness may eventually resolve, but the range of motion in the shoulder may never be completely restored.

Physical Examination

On physical examination, there may be mild wasting of the shoulder muscles. Decreased active and passive range of motion of the shoulder is noted.

■ Diagnostic Evaluation

Standard radiographs, including AP and lateral views, may reveal decreased bone density in the humerus.

■ Differential Diagnosis

- Posttraumatic stiffness
- Rotator cuff disease

■ Treatment

Nonoperative treatment is the treatment of choice and includes short-term use of nonsteroidal anti-inflammatory drugs (NSAIDs), heat, physical therapy, and daily range-of-motion exercises. Intra-articular steroids and manipulation under anesthesia may also be helpful. Capsular release via either arthroscopic or open techniques is generally reserved for cases with more severe and functionally limiting chronic symptoms.

Impingement Syndrome and Rotator Cuff Disease

It is best to consider impingement syndrome and rotator cuff disease as a spectrum of disorders spanning from irritation of the subacromial bursa to frank failure of the rotator cuff tendons. In the 1970s, Neer classified subacromial impingement into three successive stages: (1) repetitive microtrauma resulting in edema and hemorrhage in the subacromial bursa and supraspinatus tendon, which leads to (2) fibrosis and tendonitis in the distal supraspinatus tendon insertion and, eventually, (3) failure of the tendon and tearing of the rotator cuff.

Forward flexion of the humerus narrows the subacromial space and impinges on the rotator cuff and overlying bursal tissue. In young athletes, occult instability of the glenohumeral joint, bursal thickening of the rotator cuff, and contracture of the posterior capsule may result in impingement that may then progress through the stages originally described by Neer. Older patients may develop an acromial spur secondary to repeated rotator cuff injury and traction of the coracoacromial ligament.

■ Clinical Manifestations

The typical patient with impingement syndrome is younger than 40 years of age and presents with a history of sudden shoulder pain following strenuous exercise. Common inciting exercises include throwing a baseball, playing tennis, lifting weights, and painting. In most minor cases, the patient may report mild shoulder pain that becomes severe during movements that flex and/or abduct the patient's arm.

Patients who are between 40 and 50 years of age often present with either severe initial impingement syndrome or chronic impingement syndrome. The classic patient with chronic impingement syndrome will give a history of intermittent attacks controlled with NSAIDs, rest, and modified activities. The pain is often worse at night and often prevents the patient from sleeping on the affected side. The patient may further give a history of restricted ability to perform activities of daily living such as brushing hair or dressing because of shoulder pain and stiffness.

The typical patient with a partial or complete tear of the rotator cuff tendon is 40 to 50 years old and offers a history of shoulder pain refractory to NSAIDs and other treatments. The patient will usually give a history of worsening shoulder pain, stiffness, and weakness. Less commonly, a complete or partial tear of the rotator cuff will present after a sudden trauma or jerking movement of the shoulder. In this case, the patient will give a history of the trauma and recall that the pain began suddenly. Patients with rotator cuff tendon tears may not be able to abduct their arms.

Physical Examination
IMPINGEMENT SYNDROME
The Neer test is an excellent clinical examination for impingement syndrome. In this test, the examiner stabilizes the scapula with one hand and flexes the patient's shoulder with the other. By performing this maneuver, the examiner abuts the patient's greater tuberosity of the humerus onto the undersurface of the coracoacromial arch. The test is positive if the maneuver elicits pain.

Another excellent impingement test is the Hawkins test. In this test the shoulder is abducted to 90 degrees in the plane of the scapula with the elbow flexed, and then the shoulder is moved firmly into internal rotation (Figure 2-3). When this maneuver elicits pain, it is considered positive for impingement.

Perhaps the best clinical test in a patient with positive impingement signs (Neer or Hawkins) or painful range of motion is

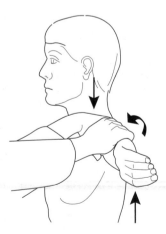

Figure 2-3 • The supraspinatus impingement test (Hawkins' test) being performed. (Reproduced with permission from Gross, J. *Musculoskeletal Examination,* second edition. Figure 8.97, p. 191. Blackwell Publishing, 2002).

to inject 10 mL of 1% lidocaine (or another anesthetic) into the subacromial space. There are multiple injection procedure approaches to deliver the anesthetic into the subacromial space. A posterolateral approach, using the acromion as an easily palpated superficial landmark, is often preferred. The impingement signs and range of motion are then tested again. If the patient has a positive Hawkins and Neer test before the anesthetic injection and a negative Hawkins and Neer test after the injection, then the test is positive for impingement syndrome. Similarly, if the patient had a painful range of motion before the injection but asymptomatic range of motion after the injection, then the test is positive. If, however, partial or complete pain persists despite the injection, an alternative diagnosis should be considered.

ROTATOR CUFF DISEASE

To assess for a rotator cuff tear, the patient is asked to slowly and smoothly lower the arm from an abducted position. This is called the drop arm test, and it is considered positive for a tear if the patient is unable to slowly lower the arm. To specifically test for a tear in the supraspinatus tendon, both shoulders are passively abducted to 90 degrees in the plane of the scapula with the thumbs pointing to the ceiling. The examiner then applies a downward force to both arms. In a patient with a supraspinatus tear, there will be weakness in abduction, particularly from 0 to 30 degrees of abduction.

To specifically test the infraspinatus and teres minor, the patient stands with elbows at the side and flexed to 90 degrees. The examiner stabilizes the patient's elbow and tests for external rotation. A tear in the infraspinatus tendon results in weakened external rotation.

To test for a subscapularis tear, Gerber's lift-off test may be used. In Gerber's lift-off test, the patient is instructed to place one hand behind the back with the palm of the hand facing in a posterior direction. The examiner then applies an anterior force against the palm as the patient resists by trying to move the hand away from the spine. A patient with a defect in the subscapularis tendon or muscle will be unable to lift the hand away from the spine.

■ Diagnostic Evaluation

Plain film radiographs, including AP, glenohumeral joint, axillary, lateral, and scapular outlet views, are all obtained in an impingement series. On the scapular outlet view, the acromion is visualized and may be categorized. Bigliani described three types of acromions (Table 2-1). Type II is the most common. Types II and III reduce the subacromial space and may be associated with increased risk of impingement syndrome and rotator cuff disease.

■ TABLE 2-1 Bigliani Classification of Acromions	
Type	Description
I	Flat
II	Curved
III	Hooked

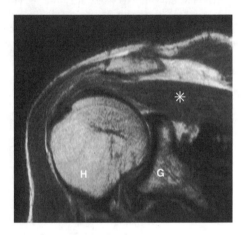

Figure 2-4 • MRI of normal rotator cuff (*) and surrounding structures. H = humerus, G = glenoid (Reproduced with permission from Gross, J. *Musculoskeletal Examination*, second edition. Figure 8.105, p. 194. Blackwell Publishing, 2002).

MRI is an excellent imaging modality for evaluating the soft tissues surrounding the shoulder (Figure 2-4). MRI is the imaging modality of choice for distinguishing between a partial-thickness rotator cuff tear and a full-thickness tear.

■ Treatment

Nonoperative conservative management is the typical initial approach to patients with impingement syndrome and/or partial-thickness tears. Modification of activities, strengthening and stretching exercises, and NSAIDs are the cornerstone of conservative care for these patients. In addition, judicious use of sub-acromial steroid injections may be particularly helpful.

In throwing athletes, loss of internal rotation secondary to posterior capsule contracture may result in exacerbation of sub-acromial impingement. Physical therapy for these patients should emphasize stretching in adduction and internal rotation.

A trial of at least 3 months of conservative care is often used before surgical intervention. In patients with evidence of a full-thickness tear, operative intervention is pursued earlier. Arthroscopic subacromial decompression has demonstrated very good results in patients with impingement syndrome, achieving satisfactory results in 80% to 90% of patients. A glenohumeral stabilization procedure may be used if occult instability of the joint is found during arthroscopy.

Careful debridement before subacromial decompression is a procedure often used for partial-thickness tears of less than 50% thickness. In full-thickness or partial-thickness tears with greater than 50% thickness involvement, repair may be accomplished through a "mini-open" or standard open technique. It is critical that after surgery, patients are enrolled in early passive range-of-motion exercises, with isometric exercises beginning around 6 weeks postop in order to avoid stiffness. Patients should be informed that structured rotator cuff strengthening exercises should be performed between 6 weeks and 3 months postop, with a return to overhead sports typically around 4 to 6 months postop.

Long Head of the Biceps Disorders

The overhead athlete may develop shoulder pain as a result of a variety of biceps tendon disorders. The tendon of the long head of the biceps is believed to serve as an anterior stabilizer of the shoulder. Recall that the short head of the biceps arises from the coracoid process and the long head of the biceps arises from the supraglenoid tubercle. Repetitive pulling on the long head of the biceps pulls on the supraglenoid tubercle and may contribute to a superior labral anterior posterior (SLAP) lesion. The biceps brachii is innervated by the musculocutaneous nerve and inserts into the radial tuberosity. When the arm is raised, the biceps tendon becomes vulnerable to impingement between the acromial arch, the coracoacromial ligament, and the humeral head.

■ Clinical Manifestations

The typical patient with bicipital tendonitis is an overhead athlete (e.g., tennis player, baseball pitcher) who presents with complaints of anterior shoulder pain that is made worse with overhead activities. The pain is usually alleviated with rest. The patient will characteristically offer a history of a forceful extension or external rotation with the arm in abduction that immediately precipitated the symptoms.

In patients with SLAP lesions, the chief complaint is typically shoulder pain, clicking, and/or popping with overhead activities, particularly throwing a ball.

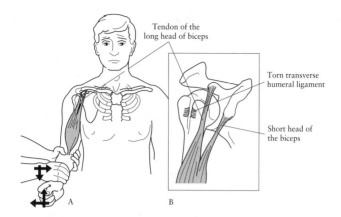

Tendon of the
long head of biceps

Torn transverse
humeral ligament

Short head of
the biceps

A   B

Figure 2-5 • (A) The Yergason test for integrity of the long head of the biceps tendon in the bicipital grove. (B) If the ligament is damaged, the biceps will sublux, as shown. (Reproduced with permission from Gross, J. *Musculoskeletal Examination,* second edition. Figure 8.95, p. 190. Blackwell Publishing, 2002).

Physical Examination

BICIPITAL TENDONITIS

Tenderness in the bicipital groove is typical of bicipital tendonitis. The Speed test is an excellent test for bicipital tendonitis. In this test, flexion of the arm with extended elbow and hand held in supination is resisted. If this maneuver produces pain, the test is considered positive for bicipital tendonitis. The Yergason test is also useful. In this test, the patient is instructed to flex the elbow to 90 degrees and then supinate the arm against resistance (Figure 2-5 A and B). The Yergason test is positive if this maneuver elicits pain that localizes to the long head of the biceps tendon.

Biceps subluxation is often found in association with subscapularis rupture and a positive Gerber lift-off test (see previous section for description of this test). Biceps instability may be tested for by palpating the biceps tendon in the groove while holding the arm in an externally rotated, abducted position. The examiner internally and externally rotates the arm. If the biceps is unstable, this maneuver may elicit a painful click as the tendon subluxes over the lesser tuberosity.

SLAP LESIONS

In SLAP lesions, both the Speed and Yergason tests may be positive. The O'Brien compression test is useful in differentiating between a SLAP lesion and AC joint disease. To perform the O'Brien test, the patient is instructed to stand and keep the elbow in full extension as the patient flexes the arm to 90 degrees. The arm is then adducted 10 to 15 degrees internally rotated such that the thumb points at the floor. Standing behind the patient, the examiner applies downward-directed force to the arms as the patient resists. With the examiner and patient in the exact same position, the maneuver is repeated, but this time with the patient's hands fully supinated. The patient has a positive O'Brien test for a SLAP lesion if the pain is worse with the first maneuver (thumbs down), and provided that the pain is experienced by the patient within the shoulder. By contrast, the test suggests AC joint disease if the pain is experienced on top of the shoulder.

■ Diagnostic Evaluation

For evaluating suspected SLAP lesions, MRI is particularly helpful. However, direct inspection and probing during arthroscopy remains the gold standard for diagnosis.

■ Treatment

Bicipital tendonitis is treated initially with NSAIDs, activity modification to avoid overhead activities, ice, and physical therapy. An injection of steroid and anesthetic may also be delivered into the bicipital groove. Caution should be used for multiple injections because of the increased risk of tendon rupture. For patients with refractory symptoms despite aggressive conservative care, surgical options include tendon debridement, acromioplasty with anterior acromionectomy, or tenodesis.

The treatment of SLAP lesions begins with conservative care, including modification of activities, and strengthening and stretching exercises. Surgical options include debridement of the frayed labrum with tendon repair of the biceps anchor, and biceps tenodesis, as necessary.

Rotator Cuff Calcific Tendonitis

Calcific tendonitis is a condition that is not unique to the shoulder. It is known to occur in the tendons and ligaments of the knee, ankle, hip, and elbow. Although it may be an asymptomatic incidental finding on radiograph, in some patients calcific tendonitis may be a source of significant morbidity. The cause of calcific tendonitis is not known but is believed to be related to local ischemia.

■ Clinical Manifestations

The typical patient is a young, active adult who presents with a complaint of pain that increases in severity with activities and decreases with rest. The patient will often report a crescendo pattern of pain beginning with activity and taking several days to subside after the activity has been stopped. The involved joint is often exquisitely tender, limiting both active and passive range of motion of the shoulder.

■ Diagnostic Evaluation

Plain film radiographs, including AP and lateral views, are indicated and will reveal a calcification, typically immediately superior to the greater tuberosity where the supraspinatus tendon inserts. The calcification may be seen to resolve on serial radiographs as the patient's symptoms improve.

■ Treatment

The primary modality of treatment is conservative and includes modification of activities, resting the arm in a sling, heat modalities, and NSAIDs. If this treatment is unsuccessful after several weeks, ultrasound-guided aspiration and lavage of the calcification has been found to be an effective minimally invasive procedure for removing the calcification and restoring function. In patients who are refractory to aspiration and lavage, surgical removal of the calcification may be performed.

Acromioclavicular Joint Injuries

AC ligaments offer the shoulder joint horizontal stability while the coracoclavicular ligaments provide vertical stability. Table 2-2 describes the six types of AC injuries. Type VI AC injury is rare.

AC injuries may result from direct acute trauma (e.g., falling onto the shoulder) or chronic repetitive microtrauma. AC injuries are particularly common in contact sports such as football, ice hockey, and rugby.

■ TABLE 2-2 Classification of AC Ligament Injuries	
Type	Description
I	Sprain of the AC ligament
II	Disruption of the AC ligament
III	Disruption of both the AC and coracoclavicular ligaments
IV	Complete dislocation of the distal clavicle with posterior displacement that penetrates the trapezius
V	Dislocation with more than 100% displacement of the distal clavicle
VI	Inferior dislocation of the distal clavicle into the subcoracoid space

■ Clinical Manifestations

The typical patient is an athlete competing in a contact sport who relates a history of direct trauma (such as a direct blow) to the acromion or else a fall onto the shoulder. The fall is often immediately followed by pain and swelling of the clavicle. In type I and II AC injuries, focal tenderness over the joint is often found. In addition, the patient often has difficulty with adducting the arm across the body. In type III injury, deformity of the AC joint may be noted in addition to tenderness.

■ Diagnostic Evaluation

Plain film radiographic evaluation, including AP, axillary, and a lateral projection of the scapula view is indicated. An AP weight-bearing projection may also be indicated. X-ray will reveal no displacement of the clavicle in type I injuries, up to 50% displacement of the clavicle with an increase in the coracoclavicular distance in type II injuries, and 50% to 100% displacement of the clavicle in type III injuries.

■ Treatment

Type I and type II AC injuries are treated with conservative management, including ice, pain medications as needed, and a shoulder sling. Physical therapy with range-of-motion and strengthening exercises is gradually implemented as tolerated by the patient. Symptoms that are refractory to conservative care may necessitate a distal clavicle resection with formal coracoclavicular stabilization.

Type III treatment is often the same as for type I and II injuries. However, patients often complain of cosmetic deformity with conservative care for a type III AC injury. Many physicians advocate surgical correction of a type III injury, particularly in patients with active lifestyles. Surgical correction of a type III AC injury involves coracoclavicular fixation with screws, or distal clavicle resection with transfer to the coracoacromial ligament and stabilization of the coracoclavicular interval with suture, soft tissue, or hardware.

Type IV, V, and VI AC injuries are treated with surgery, including coracoclavicular internal fixation and/or AC fixation. Postoperatively, these patients require up to 6 weeks in a sling in order to prevent displacement. After approximately 6 weeks, a structured range-of-motion and strengthening exercise program is begun.

Clavicular Fracture

Clavicular fractures are the most common type of fracture in childhood. They account for 35% of all fractures in the shoulder and 4% to 5% of all fractures. Eighty-five percent of clavicular fractures involve the middle third of the clavicle. During childbirth, the clavicle is the most frequently fractured bone.

■ Clinical Manifestations

A patient will typically report a fall onto an outstretched arm. The clavicle will be painful and swollen, and the patient may report decreased range of motion in the arm.

Physical Examination
On exam, the patient's clavicle is tender and swollen. Active and passive range of motion of the shoulder is decreased. Because the clavicle is such a superficial structure, the bony defect may be palpated.

■ Diagnostic Evaluation

Plain film radiographs, including AP and cephalic tilt views, should be obtained.

■ Treatment

The initial treatment of most clavicular fractures is a figure-eight bandage or arm sling. As soon as patient comfort permits, the bandage or sling is removed and range-of-motion exercises are initiated. Radiographic evidence of healing is usually seen at approximately 6 weeks with return to full function at 12 weeks.

When the clavicular fracture is open, or when the fracture is displaced with impending skin or neurovascular compromise, open reduction with internal fixation is performed.

Clavicular fractures in neonates are treated with immobilization of the fracture for 10 to 12 weeks.

■ Complications

Brachial plexus injuries may result. Neurovascular compromise of surrounding structures is a rare complication.

Humeral Shaft Fracture

Humeral shaft fractures account for 3% of all fractures. Direct trauma is the cause of most fractures.

■ Clinical Manifestations

Typically, the patient will relate a history of direct trauma to the arm. Elderly patients may fracture the humerus after falling. Pain and swelling are typical of humeral fractures.

Physical Examination

It is critical to perform a thorough exam to assess motor and sensory function of the radial, median, and ulnar nerves. This exam serves as a baseline for future exams to detect potential neurovascular compromise as the patient is treated. See the High-Yield Surgical and Functional Anatomy section in the Elbow and Forearm chapter for discussion of how to clinically assess median, ulnar, and radial nerves.

■ Diagnostic Evaluation

Standard AP and lateral views of the humerus should be obtained.

■ Treatment

A coaptation splint, collar and cuff, or hanging cast may be used to nonsurgically manage most patients with humeral shaft fractures. Patients should be instructed to remain upright as much as possible and to not lean on their elbow. Initial immobilization of the arm may be weaned as pain decreases. The arm is then placed in a functional brace, and range-of-motion exercises may follow.

Open humeral fractures, brachial plexus injuries, vascular injuries, fractures that extend to the elbow, and fractures that are not adequately aligned with nonsurgical intervention are all indications for surgical intervention. Surgical options include plates and screws and intramedullary nailing of the humeral shaft fracture. Early use of crutches following plate-and-screw stabilization is important to maximize function.

■ Complications

Radial nerve injuries have been reported in as many as 18% of patients. Most radial nerve injuries (more than 90%) resolve within 3 to 4 months. Progressive neurologic symptoms may require an exploration to rule out entrapment.

3

Elbow and Forearm

High-Yield Surgical and Functional Anatomy

The elbow is a hinge type of synovial joint designed to allow functional movement of the forearm and hand in space. The elbow joint is made up of three articulations: (1) the humeroulnar joint is the largest and most stable elbow articulation, relying on the medial collateral ligament for its stability; (2) the humeroradial joint is composed of the radial head and the capitellum of the humerus and rotates during supination and pronation; and (3) the proximal radioulnar joint is held together by the annular ligament.

There are numerous surgical approaches to the elbow joint and surrounding structures, including anterior, posterior, medial, anterolateral, and posterolateral approaches. Because the important neurovascular structures pass the elbow joint on the anterior and posterior aspects of the joint, medial and lateral approaches to the elbow are safe but offer relatively limited exposure. By contrast, the posterior approach provides the best overall exposure but risks injuring important structures such as the ulnar nerve and radial nerve.

■ Anterior and Anterolateral Approaches

The anterior approach to the elbow is used primarily to repair injuries to the median nerve, brachial artery, radial nerve, and biceps tendon. The anterolateral approach is used for open reduction and internal fixation of the capitellum, treatment of biceps avulsion from the radial tuberosity, and other pathologies. In the anterior elbow, the biceps tendon is easily palpated as a taut band during resisted flexion. In the anterior elbow, the median nerve runs lateral to the brachial artery. Injury to the median nerve at this point may result in loss of forearm pronation, wrist and digit flexion, and thumb apposition. In addition, a loss of sensation may result on the lateral portion of the palm, including the palmar surface of the first three digits.

The brachial artery is a continuation of the axillary artery and is the chief blood supplier to the arm. The brachial divides into the radial and ulnar arteries. Injury to the brachial artery represents a surgical emergency.

The musculocutaneous nerve terminates in the lateral antebrachial cutaneous nerve at the lateral border of the tendon of the biceps. This nerve supplies the skin of the forearm.

The radial nerve is the largest branch of the brachial plexus and enters the arm posterior to the brachial artery. It is identified crossing the anterior elbow in the intermuscular groove of the brachialis and brachioradialis muscles. Injury to the radial nerve characteristically results in the clinical sign of wrist drop.

■ Posterior Approach

The posterior approach to the elbow is primarily used for open reduction and internal fixation of distal humerus fractures, removal of loose bodies from the elbow joint, and treating nonunions of the distal humerus. The superficial bony olecranon process at the proximal end of the ulna is easily palpated when the elbow is kept in a flexed position. The ulnar nerve typically runs in the bony groove posterior to the medial epicondyle. Injury to the ulnar nerve may result in an inability to adduct or abduct the last four digits. The triceps inserts into the proximal portion of the olecranon and is innervated by the radial nerve. The function of the triceps is to extend the forearm.

Lateral and Medial Epicondylitis

For decades the term "tennis elbow" has been used to describe a gamut of symptoms involving the elbow. In fact, in order to be specific, the term "tennis elbow" should be reserved to describe tendonitis of the forearm muscle tendons that insert into the lateral epicondyle of the humerus. The term "golfer's elbow" is often used to describe medial epicondylitis.

Repetitive pronation and supination of the forearm is believed to instigate small tears at the origin of the extensor carpi radialis brevis and/or the extensor carpi radialis longus and/or the extensor carpi ulnaris that leads to lateral epicondylitis. Repetitive forearm pronation with the wrist in flexion predisposes to medial epicondylitis, which is much less common than lateral epicondylitis. It should be noted, however, that recent studies suggest that inflammation may not play a central role in medial or lateral epicondylitis, making the names potential misnomers.

■ Clinical Manifestations

The typical patient with lateral epicondylitis is between 30 and 50 years old and participates in a racquet or throwing sport, or has a job or hobby such as plumbing or carpentry. All of these activities share the common feature of involving repetitive pronation and supination of the forearm. The patient will typically complain of pain over the lateral epicondyle. The pain is exacerbated by activity. As the disease progresses, the intensity of the pain increases and even actions such as pouring tea, shaking hands, or grasping objects become difficult.

The typical patient with medial epicondylitis is also between 30 and 50 years of age and often participates in a sport such as golf, in which there is repetitive forearm pronation with wrist flexion. The patient will characteristically complain of pain over the medial epicondyle.

Physical Examination

On physical examination, the elbow appears normal on inspection. In lateral epicondylitis, the lateral epicondyle is tender to palpation. In medial epicondylitis, the medial epicondyle is tender to palpation.

Patients with lateral epicondylitis have reproducible symptoms with resisted wrist extension. The Cozen test is a useful examination technique to perform. In this test, the patient's elbow is stabilized and the patient makes a fist, pronates the arm, and radially deviates the wrist against resistance. If the patient experiences a sharp, sudden, severe pain over the lateral epicondyle, the test is positive for lateral epicondylitis.

Patients with medial epicondylitis have reproducible symptoms with resisted forearm pronation and wrist flexion.

■ Diagnostic Evaluation

Plain film radiography is often normal but may show calcification at the tendon insertion. Magnetic resonance imaging (MRI) is not routinely indicated but if obtained will demonstrate tendon thickening with increased T1 and T2 signals.

■ Treatment

Conservative treatment is the mainstay of therapy for lateral epicondylitis. Conservative modalities for lateral epicondylitis include physical therapy with strengthening and stretching exercises, use of a counterforce brace, ultrasound, electrical stimulation, and/or iontophoresis. Additional conservative modalities include icing and/or steroid injections. In more than 95% of patients, conservative therapy achieves satisfactory results. The remaining refractory cases may be treated either surgically under local anesthesia with percutaneous release of the extensor origin, with arthroscopic release of the extensor carpi radialis brevis, or open debridement.

Medial epicondylitis is treated conservatively in a similar manner to lateral epicondylitis, but the results are less satisfactory. Surgical options include release of the flexor pronator origin, excision of the pathologic tissue, and reattachment of the flexor pronator origin. When patients present with preoperative ulnar nerve symptoms, decompression and transposition of the nerve should be performed at the time of operation.

Ulnar Collateral Ligament Injury

Overhead athletes, and pitchers in particular, are especially susceptible to elbow injuries. Pitching biomechanics may be divided into six successive stages: (1) the windup, (2) early cocking, (3) late cocking, (4) acceleration, (5) deceleration, and (6) the follow-through. During the late cocking and acceleration phases, excessive valgus forces are generated across the medial elbow. Repetitive excessive valgus forces may lead to ulnar collateral ligament injury primarily of the anterior band.

■ Clinical Manifestations

The typical patient is a baseball pitcher or other athlete who participates in overhead sports and complains of acute or chronic medial elbow pain and tenderness that is made worse with continued overhead activity. Often, the patient will also complain of associated ulnar nerve symptoms such as radiating pain, numbness, and/or tingling in the ring and little finger.

Physical Examination

On physical examination, the ulnar collateral ligament is tender. One-quarter to one-half of patients will demonstrate clinical laxity in response to a valgus stress applied by the examiner.

■ Diagnostic Evaluation

Standard plain film radiography should be ordered, including anteroposterior (AP), lateral, axial, and valgus stress views. Contrast MRI is routinely ordered. Early in the course of the injury, MRI will show low signal intensity on T1-weighted images and no changes in T2. As the injury progresses and becomes more chronic and severe, fluid on T2-weighted images may be detected and represent a partially or completely detached fragment.

■ Treatment

For most patients the initial treatment approach is conservative, utilizing strengthening and range-of-motion exercises. However, for competitive athletes who are hoping to return to competition, surgical intervention is required. The surgical option often used is reconstruction of the ligament with a palmaris longus tendon graft woven in a figure-eight pattern. For patients with concomitant ulnar nerve involvement, the nerve should be subcutaneously transposed. Approximately 80% of athletes are able to return to competition within 1 year.

Osteochondritis Dissecans

Osteochondritis dissecans (OCD) is a condition in which a fragment of cartilage and subchondral bone separates from an intact articular surface. The fragment may completely or incompletely separate. OCD in the elbow occurs primarily in the capitellum. As with OCD in the knee and ankle, the pathophysiology of OCD in the elbow is multifactorial and includes repetitive trauma and ischemia. In overhead athletes, repetitive abnormally high valgus stresses place severe compressive forces on the lateral aspect of the elbow between the radial head and the capitellum, potentially initiating osteochondritic changes.

■ Clinical Manifestations

The typical patient is about 12 years old and plays a sport such as baseball or tennis. The patient presents with a complaint of insidious onset of generalized elbow pain, swelling, and intermittent range-of-motion restriction. The symptoms are typically exacerbated by movement and relieved by rest. Occasionally, patients will be able to point to a singular traumatic incident that precipitated the symptoms. Patients with loose body lesions may also complain of locking, catching, or giving way of the elbow.

Physical Examination

On physical examination, the elbow will usually be diffusely swollen, and there may be tenderness over the capitellum. Range of motion may be slightly limited. In patients with loose body lesions, locking or catching may be present.

■ Diagnostic Evaluation

Plain film radiographs, including AP, lateral, and oblique views of the elbow, should be obtained. MRI and/or computed tomography (CT) is also useful in defining the extent of the lesion. MRI is more sensitive than plain film radiographs and is particularly useful in preoperative planning. When MRI is contraindicated, CT is a good second alternative.

■ Treatment

Patients with mild to moderate disease should be treated with at least 8 to 12 weeks of conservative therapy, consisting of activity modification, bracing, range-of-motion exercises, and nonsteroidal anti-inflammatory drugs (NSAIDs). Severe disease and mild to moderate disease that does not respond to conservative care may be considered for surgical intervention. Arthroscopic lesion removal and abrasion chrondroplasty has shown some preliminary positive results. However, the results of surgery for elbow OCD have been mixed overall, often resulting in decreased range of motion and occasionally decreased function.

Cubital Tunnel Syndrome

Cubital tunnel syndrome is a nonspecific term used to describe compression or entrapment neuropathy of the ulnar nerve at the elbow. Cubital tunnel syndrome is the second most common peripheral neuropathy, second only to carpal tunnel syndrome.

The ulnar nerve travels behind the medial epicondyle through a fibro-osseous canal en route from the arm to the forearm. There are many potential specific sites of compression as the nerve passes the elbow, notably between the two heads of the flexor carpi ulnaris. Other sites for potential compression include a space-occupying lesion such as a ganglion cyst, the arcade of Struthers, medial intermuscular septum, and beneath Osborne's ligament.

■ Clinical Manifestations

The typical patient in the beginning phase of the syndrome presents with a complaint of a deep aching sensation. As cubital syndrome progresses, the patient may report paresthesias in the ring and little fingers. Later in the syndrome, the patient may note loss of fine motor control in the fourth and fifth fingers, and finally loss of fourth and fifth finger flexion. The patient will report increased symptoms with elbow flexion. An important question to ask the patient is whether the dorsum of the ring and little finger are numb or tingling. When there is no paresthesia present in the dorsum of the ring and little finger, compression of the ulnar nerve at the wrist is implicated, not the elbow, because the ulnar nerve branches proximal to the wrist into a dorsal sensory branch being innervated by the dorsal fourth and fifth fingers. If compression occurs in the wrist, the dorsal side of the fourth and fifth fingers will be spared.

In severe cubital tunnel syndrome, the patient may also complain of severe medial elbow pain. Even in severe disease, however, nocturnal symptoms that wake the patient are much less common than in carpal tunnel syndrome.

Physical Examination

One-quarter of asymptomatic patients will have a positive Tinel's sign. In this test, the nerve is tapped repetitively as it passes superficially through the tunnel. The sign is positive when the tapping reproduces the symptoms. This test is sensitive but non-specific for cubital tunnel syndrome. Another test is to flex the elbow maximally, put the forearm into supination and the wrist in slight extension, and have the patient hold that position for 60 seconds. Unfortunately, because close to one-quarter of asymptomatic people also have a false-positive result from this test, this test is also nonspecific. Finally, fifth digit abduction weakness is the Wartenberg's sign for cubital tunnel syndrome.

■ Diagnostic Evaluation

Electrodiagnostic nerve conduction studies are very helpful in establishing the diagnosis.

■ Treatment

Conservative management is the first line of therapy for patients with mild to moderate symptoms. Conservative care includes splinting the elbow at 45 degrees, padding the nerve, and activity modification to avoid positions of the elbow that exacerbate symptoms. Steroid injections for this condition are highly ineffective because there is no tenosynovium for the steroids to reduce inflammation. In patients with more severe, functionally limiting symptoms or patients with refractory mild to moderate disease, surgical intervention should be considered. When surgery is undertaken, it is important to eliminate all sites of compression. In situ decompression may be considered for mild disease and a nonsubluxating nerve. In moderate to severe disease, an anterior submuscular transposition should be undertaken.

Outcome from surgery is best predicted by the presence or absence of preexisting intrinsic muscle atrophy, with the presence and degree of intrinsic atrophy correlating closely with poor outcome.

■ Complications

Incomplete nerve decompression or perineural scarring are the most common causes of complications from this procedure, which is usually well tolerated. The medial antebrachial cutaneous nerve may be injured and result in a painful scar.

Distal Humeral Shaft Fracture

Distal humeral shaft fractures have a bimodal age distribution. In younger populations, they tend to occur as a result of high-energy trauma such as from a motor vehicle accident. In older patient populations, they may occur as a result of a small fall. Patients present with pain and swelling.

Physical Examination

A careful neurovascular examination is particularly important to perform in patients with presumed distal humeral shaft fractures.

■ **Diagnostic Evaluation**

Traction AP and lateral radiographs are necessary before surgery because the fragments generally overlap with regular AP and lateral films.

■ **Treatment**

If the fracture is displaced, open reduction with rigid internal fixation that allows for early range of motion is necessary for optimal recovery. This is usually accomplished with a lag screw and neutralization plate fixation in two different planes: one posterior on the radial column and one medial on the ulnar column.

In patients with comorbidities who are elderly, a comminuted distal humeral fracture is difficult to treat with open reduction and internal fixation, and primary total elbow arthroplasty may be offered as an alternative option.

For most patients, prognosis is best predicted by the extent of concomitant soft tissue damage. Because high-energy traumas tend to have the greatest involvement of the soft tissues, they tend to have worse outcome compared to lower-energy traumas.

■ **Complications**

Failure of fixation, malunion, nonunion, olecranon osteotomy nonunion, painful hardware, infection, and ulnar nerve damage are all potential complications.

Supracondylar Fracture

Supracondylar fractures are the most common type of pediatric elbow fracture and account for 10% of all pediatric fractures (Figure 3-1). Gartland classified supracondylar fractures (Table 3-1).

■ **Clinical Manifestations**

The typical patient is a child who has suffered an extension type of injury from a fall onto an outstretched hand. On physical examination, the elbow is tender and swollen. An anterior interosseous nerve injury can be evaluated for by having the patient make the "okay" sign with the finger and thumb. Patients with an anterior interossus nerve injury will be unable to completely perform this sign.

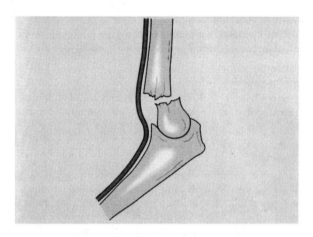

Figure 3-1 • Supracondylar fracture of the humerus. (Reproduced with permission from Duckworth, T. *Lecture Notes on Orthopaedics and Fractures,* third edition. Figure 15.2, p. 107. Blackwell Publishing, 1995).

■ TABLE 3-1   Gartland Classification of Supracondylar Fractures

Type	Description
I	Nondisplaced
II	Anterior gapping, some rotational malalignment, and an intact posterior hinge
III	Loss of all cortex continuity

■ Diagnostic Evaluation

Plain film radiographs, including AP, lateral, and oblique apical views, should be obtained.

■ Treatment

A long arm cast is used to treat Gartland type I fractures. Percutaneous pinning is usually used to treat Gartland type II fractures. Type III fractures and some type II fractures are treated with closed reduction with smooth Kirschner wires. If the surgeon decides an open reduction is necessary, the approach is always from the side that is opposite the direction of the displacement of the distal fragment. This is done in order to remove pressure from the remaining periosteum.

■ Complications

When an anterior interosseous nerve injury is sustained, the patient can be reassured that most such complications spontaneously resolve within 3 to 4 months. Ulnar nerve injury is also a complication.

Radial Head Fracture

Radial head fractures account for as much as 30% of all elbow fractures and are commonly associated with ligamentous injury. Table 3-2 describes the four types of radial head fractures.

■ Clinical Manifestations

The patient will complain of pain and swelling at the lateral elbow. On physical examination, the lateral aspect of the elbow will be tender and swollen.

■ Diagnostic Evaluation

Standard plain film radiographs, including AP, lateral, and oblique views of the elbow and radiocapitella, should be obtained.

■ Treatment

Type I radial head fractures that are not displaced or type II fractures that are minimally displaced less than 2 mm are treated conservatively with early range-of-motion and strengthening exercises. Type II fractures with greater than 2 mm of displacement or with mechanical block, type III, and type IV fractures are treated with open reduction and internal fixation. Additionally, if the medial collateral ligament is found to have instability, it should be repaired during surgery.

■ Complications

Decreased range of motion and posterior interosseous nerve injury are possible complications.

■ TABLE 3-2	Classification of Radial Head Fractures
Type	Description
I	Nondisplaced
II	Single displaced fracture
III	Comminuted fracture
IV	Radial head fracture with elbow dislocation

Monteggia Fracture

The Monteggia fracture is characterized by a proximal ulnar fracture and radial head dislocation (Figure 3-2). The most common classification of Monteggia fractures is by Bado (Table 3-3). Type I is the most common Monteggia fracture, and type II is the second most common.

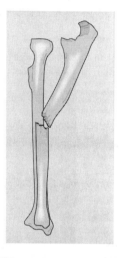

Figure 3-2 • Monteggia fracture of the ulna (dislocation of radial head). (Reproduced with permission from Duckworth, T. *Lecture Notes on Orthopaedics and Fractures,* third edition. Figure 15.9, p. 114. Blackwell Publishing, 1995).

▣ TABLE 3-3	Bado Classification of Monteggia Fractures
Type	**Description**
I	Anterior radial head is dislocated along with an apex anterior proximal one-third ulna fracture
II	Posterior head dislocation and apex posterior proximal one-third ulna fracture
III	Lateral head dislocation and proximal ulnar metaphysal fracture
IV	Anterior radial head dislocation with a proximal one-third radius and ulna fracture

■ Clinical Manifestations

The typical patient describes a history of falling onto an outstretched hand. On physical examination, there is usually obvious ulnar deformity. The lateral elbow is tender.

■ Diagnostic Evaluation

Plain film radiographs, including AP and lateral views of the elbow and wrist, are indicated.

■ Treatment

Closed reduction may be used in children depending on the severity. Types I, III, and IV Monteggia fractures are each treated with open reduction and internal fixation and then put in a cast with 110 degrees of flexion. Type II fracture is treated with open reduction and internal fixation and then put in a cast with 70 degrees of flexion.

■ Complications

The posterior interosseous nerve may be injured and results in weakened wrist extensors. When present, this nerve injury usually heals spontaneously.

4

Wrist and Hand

High-Yield Surgical and Functional Anatomy

The anatomy of the hand and wrist is as complex and intricate as its function. The anatomy is best approached via the different surgical approaches. The hand and wrist may be approached from the volar or dorsal aspect.

■ Dorsal Approach

The dorsal approach to the wrist is used for wrist fusion, open reduction and internal fixation of distal radial and carpal fractures, and other pathologies. Many vital structures traverse the dorsal aspect of the wrist. Most superficial, from radius to ulna, is the superficial branch of the radial nerve, cephalic vein, basilic vein, and the dorsal cutaneous branch of the ulnar never. Deep to these structures is the extensor retinaculum. The extensor retinaculum is a fibrous band of tissue that forms six tunnels from the wrist to the hand. Each of these tunnels transmits tendons of the extensor muscles. In the first tunnel are the tendons of the abductor pollicis longus and extensor pollicis brevis tendons. In the second tunnel are the tendons of the extensor carpi radialis longus and extensor carpi radialis brevis muscles. In the third tunnel is the tendon of the extensor pollicis longus muscle. In the fourth tunnel are the tendons of the extensor digitorum and extensor indicis muscles. In the fifth tunnel is the tendon of the extensor digiti minimi muscle. In the sixth tunnel is the tendon of the extensor carpi ulnaris muscle. All of the muscles with tendons passing through the dorsal tunnels are innervated by the radial nerve.

On the lateral aspect of the wrist is the anatomic snuff box. This box refers to the triangular skin depression bounded by the extensor pollicis longus tendon medially and the tendons of the abductor pollicis longus and extensor pollicis brevis laterally. The radial artery also passes this location deep to the tendons. The anatomic snuff box is an important anatomic landmark because the scaphoid bone can be palpated in the floor.

■ **Volar Approach**

The volar approach to the wrist is used for decompression of the median nerve, open reduction and internal fixation of distal radial fractures, drainage of midpalmar sepsis, decompression of ulnar nerve entrapment in the tunnel of Guyon, and other pathologies. The superficial landmarks include the thenar crease and the tendon of the palmaris longus muscle (absent in approximately 10% of the population), which (when present) is best palpated by having the patient flex the wrist and pinch all the fingers together. The carpal bones form the concave base of the carpal tunnel, and the strong flexor retinaculum forms the roof. Several vital structures are found superficial to the flexor retinaculum.

The flexor carpi ulnaris muscle arises from the medial epicondyle of the humerus. Its tendon is a superficial volar structure that inserts onto the pisiform bone. The flexor carpi ulnaris is innervated by the ulnar nerve, and its function is to flex and adduct the hand.

The ulnar nerve is superficial to the flexor retinaculum. The ulnar nerve runs lateral to the pisiform bone through the tunnel of Guyon, which is a site of potential entrapment. The ulnar artery runs lateral to the ulnar nerve. The palmar cutaneous branch of the median nerve has a variable course and passes superficial to the flexor retinaculum.

Deep to the flexor retinaculum is the carpal tunnel. Through the carpal tunnel run the nine tendons to the digits and the median nerve. Each of the last four digits has two tendons. One tendon serves the flexor digitorum superficialis and one tendon serves the flexor digitorum profundus. The flexor digitorum superficialis flexes the proximal interphalangeal (PIP) joint. The flexor digitorum profundii work in unison (one tendon cannot flex without all the profundus tendons flexing) to flex the distal interphalangeal (DIP) joints. In addition, the flexor pollicis longus runs through the carpal tunnel and flexes the distal phalanx of the first digit. These tendons run posterior to the tendons through the carpal tunnel.

Carpal Tunnel Syndrome

Carpal tunnel syndrome is the most common peripheral neuropathy. Eighty-seven percent of carpal tunnel syndrome cases are bilateral. Women account for nearly 80% of all cases. The mean age at diagnosis is 51.

The carpal tunnel is a rigid structure surrounded on three sides by wrist bones and anteriorly by the dense transverse carpal ligament. Any increase in volume of the tissues or fluid within the confines of this rigid passageway increases the pressure, which decreases capillary circulation and induces ischemia in the median nerve, leading to the symptoms of carpal tunnel syndrome.

The carpal tunnel may experience increased volume loads for several reasons. Repetitive stress from combined wrist and finger flexion mechanically increases the pressure. Increased volume related to fluid retention during the third trimester in pregnancy probably accounts for the increased incidence of carpal tunnel syndrome during pregnancy. Swelling from a distal radius fracture, rheumatoid tenosynovitis, or myxedema are among the other causes of increased volume in the tunnel.

■ Clinical Manifestations

A typical patient with carpal tunnel syndrome is a woman around 50 years of age who may have a history of rheumatoid arthritis, diabetes mellitus, or hypothyroidism. The patient usually has a job or hobby that includes typing, knitting, driving long distances, or any other repetitive activity that involves simultaneous wrist and finger flexion. Early in the disease, the patient will typically complain of a vague aching sensation in the wrist with tingling, burning, and/or numbness in the first, second, and/or third digits. Sometimes the fourth digit is also involved. In some patients the aching sensation in the wrist radiates up to the neck.

As the disease progresses, symptoms of paresthesias that awaken the patient from sleep are the most sensitive predictor of carpal tunnel syndrome. Nighttime symptoms are also most reliably relieved by surgical release. It is thought that the nighttime symptoms may be related to a redistribution of extracellular water during recumbency. Also, patients may have a tendency to sleep with their hands and wrists in flexion, contributing to nighttime symptoms.

The patient may also complain of finger and hand weakness. As the disease continues to progress, the patient may lose the ability to abduct the thumb, and the patient may begin to complain of clumsiness in the hand.

Physical Examination

On physical examination, inspection may reveal wasting of the thenar muscles. Sensation testing should be performed in the median nerve distribution and compared with the little finger on the same hand and also with the opposite hand. Tinel's sign is the most *specific* test for carpal tunnel syndrome. In this test, the examiner gently repetitively taps over the course of the median nerve as it travels through the tunnel (Figure 4-1). When this tapping elicits paresthesias in the median nerve distribution, the test is positive. The compression test is the most *sensitive* test for

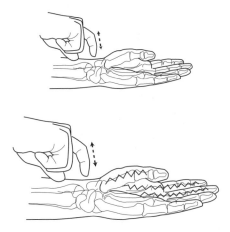

Figure 4-1 • Testing Tinel's sign at the wrist for carpal tunnel syndrome. (Reproduced with permission from Gross, J. *Musculoskeletal Examination,* second edition. Figure 10.93, p. 282. Blackwell Publishing, 2002).

carpal tunnel syndrome. In this test, pressure is applied by the examiner onto the patient's carpal tunnel, and this position is held for 60 seconds. When paresthesias are elicited in the median nerve distribution, this test is positive. Phalen's test may also be performed. In this test, both of the patient's wrists are put into flexion against one another, and this position is held for 60 seconds (Figure 4-2). The test is positive if it produces paresthesias in the median nerve distribution.

■ Diagnostic Evaluation

Although not always necessary for the diagnosis, electrodiagnostic interrogation is extremely helpful in establishing the diagnosis of carpal tunnel syndrome either before surgery or when the diagnosis is in doubt.

■ Treatment

Conservative treatment is the first line of therapy. Activity modification and splinting are cornerstones of conservative care. Patients should be taught to keep their wrists in a neutral position while typing and performing other activities that exacerbate symptoms. Splinting is also important for this purpose. Depending on the severity of symptoms, patients may initially try wearing the splints only at night. If this is unsuccessful in relieving daytime symptoms, the patients may need to wear the splint all day as well.

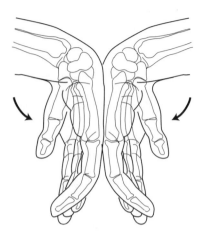

Figure 4-2 • Phalen's test. This position is held for at least 60 seconds. (Reproduced with permission from Gross, J. *Musculoskeletal Examination,* second edition. Figure 10.94, p. 283. Blackwell Publishing, 2002).

Steroid injections have been shown to relieve symptoms temporarily in up to 80% of patients. However, only 22% of patients will continue to be symptom-free at 12 months after a steroid injection.

For patients refractory to conservative care, carpal tunnel release is very successful in relieving symptoms and restoring function. Evidence suggests that the earlier the surgical intervention, the better the outcome. Endoscopic techniques have been shown to be as successful as open procedures that use larger incisions. Following surgery, splinting is unnecessary before returning to full function.

■ Complications

The primary complication of surgical intervention is a failure to achieve symptom relief. This failure is typically related to an incomplete division of the transverse carpal tunnel ligament during surgery, unrecognized proximal median nerve entrapment, severe or persistent compression, worker's compensation, and increased age.

De Quervain's Tenosynovitis

Entrapment of the abductor pollicis longus and extensor pollicis brevis tendons as they pass through the first dorsal compartment of the wrist beneath the extensor retinaculum at the radial styloid is called de Quervain's tenosynovitis. De Quervain's tenosynovitis is the second most common tendon entrapment (after trigger finger) at the hand and wrist.

■ Clinical Manifestations

The typical patient is a female between the ages of 40 and 50. The patient's chief complaint is radial side wrist pain that is typically brought on by a novel activity such as gardening.

Physical Examination

On physical examination, tenderness is appreciated over the tip of the radial styloid. Swelling may also be present at the radial styloid. The patient is often instructed to abduct the thumb as the examiner applies resistance. If this maneuver is painful for the patient, it is indicative of de Quervain's tenosynovitis. Another good test is Finkelstein's test. In this test, the patient's thumb is passively adducted across the palm with the wrist in ulnar deviation (Figure 4-3). When this maneuver produces pain at the radial styloid process, the test is considered positive.

■ Diagnostic Evaluation

No imaging is necessary in uncomplicated cases.

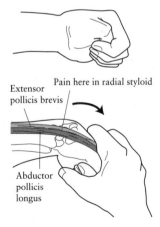

Pain here in radial styloid

Extensor
pollicis brevis

Abductor
pollicis
longus

Figure 4-3 • Finkelstein's test is used to diagnose tenosynovitis of the first dorsal compartment of the wrist, which includes the extensor pollicis and abductor pollicis longus muscles. (Reproduced with permission from Gross, J. *Musculoskeletal Examination,* second edition. Figure 10.99, p. 284. Blackwell Publishing, 2002).

■ **Treatment**

Often, the only treatment necessary is reassurance and avoidance of the offending activity. Splinting may also be useful. Corticosteroid and anesthetic injections have been used with great success for de Quervain's tenosynovitis. If symptoms persist or recur after 1 month, a second steroid and anesthetic injection may be given. After one to two steroid and anesthetic injections into the tendon sheath, 90% to 95% of patients achieve satisfactory results. However, great care must be taken when injecting steroid into this location. If the steroid is injected subcutaneously and not into the sheath, skin hypopigmentation may result.

For persistent symptoms despite conservative treatment, surgical unroofing of the first dorsal compartment should be performed. This procedure also must be done with great care in order to avoid injuring the radial nerve.

Stenosing Tenosynovitis

Trigger finger is the name given to stenosing tenosynovitis of the digital flexor tendons. The term "trigger finger" refers to the characteristic snapping observed when the patient actively flexes or extends the interphalangeal joints. Trigger finger is the most common tendon entrapment in the hand and wrist.

Stenosing tenosynovitis is caused by a slight enlargement of the tendon that causes it to fail to glide smoothly through the proximal end of the fibro-osseous tendon sheath. This enlargement of the tendon causes it to catch and give way (instead of glide) as it moves in and out of the proximal sheath.

■ **Clinical Manifestations**

The typical patient is a woman who complains of her finger "clicking" or "triggering" when she bends and extends it. The patient may or may not experience pain with the triggering. The triggering may occur on any finger, although the ring and middle fingers are most commonly involved. Often the patient will also have a history of carpal tunnel syndrome, de Quervain's tenosynovitis, or a history of a resolved trigger finger.

Physical Examination

A tender nodule may be palpated on the affected sheath. When the patient makes a fist, the involved finger snaps into place. When the patient unclenches the hand, the involved finger remains bent. It is only with a slightly increased effort that the finger snaps back into an extended position. Passive range of motion is smooth, painless, and complete.

■ Treatment

Steroid injection into the sheath is very effective at breaking the cycle of inflammation and reducing symptoms. When symptoms do not completely resolve, or if they recur, a second steroid injection may be performed after 1 month. Treating patients with one to two steroid injections provides approximately 95% of patients with resolution of symptoms. Splinting may also be helpful for these patients, either alone or in conjunction with the steroid injection(s).

For the remaining 5% with refractory symptoms, surgical trigger finger release under local anesthesia is performed. It is critical that the patient begin active range of motion with the finger immediately after surgery in order to prevent tendon adhesions at the surgical site.

Digital nerve laceration during surgery is a known potential complication. Particular care must be taken when operating on the thumb because of the proximity of the nerve to the constricting tendon sheath.

Rheumatoid Arthritis

The hand and wrist are commonly affected by rheumatoid arthritis with resulting serious morbidity. Tenosynovitis may lead to such complications as tendon rupture, erosion of the radiocarpal and intercarpal joints, and instability.

■ Clinical Manifestations

The typical patient is a woman with a preexisting history of rheumatoid arthritis presenting with pain and swelling on the ulnar side of her wrist. As the disease progresses, the patient may note increasing pain, deformity, decreasing grip strength and dexterity, and increased ulnar deviation of the wrist.

Physical Examination

On physical examination, the patient will have other signs of rheumatoid arthritis. Ulnar deviation of the wrist may be present and represents significant rheumatoid arthritis. Patients may also have a swan-neck deformity in which there is hyperextension of the PIP joint and flexion of the DIP joint. Patients may also demonstrate a boutonniere deformity in which there is flexion of the PIP joint and hyperextension of the DIP joint.

■ Diagnostic Evaluation

Plain film radiographs should be obtained and reveal characteristic findings (Figure 4-4).

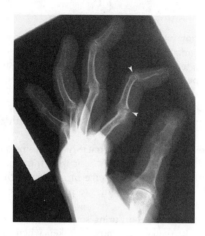

Figure 4-4 • Rheumatoid arthritis. Classis swan-neck deformity of the hands. Hyperextension of PIP joint and hyperflexion of DIP joint. (Courtesy of Cedars-Sinai Medical Center, Los Angeles, California).

■ Treatment

Treating rheumatoid arthritis of the wrist and hands is similar to treating rheumatoid arthritis of other joints. The first intervention is to treat the underlying disease. When necessary, surgical reconstruction is intended to decrease pain, increase function, and prevent deformity. Several surgical options are available for treating severely arthritic wrists. A recent study found that patients with fused wrists had greater satisfaction after surgery than those with nonfused wrists. However, other studies have shown that wrist arthroplasty yields superior results, probably because of improved dexterity of the wrists.

Ganglion

A ganglion in the musculoskeletal system is defined as a spherical accumulation of fluid produced from an adjacent tendon sheath or capsule. Women are affected twice as often as men. In contrast to a neoplasm, a ganglion is *acellular*. Although it is also a collection of clear, viscous fluid, in contrast to a cyst a ganglion is not contained in an endothelial cavity.

A ganglion in the musculoskeletal system pushes away the normal adventitial tissue and forms a pseudocyst of hyaluronic acid. The most common locations of a ganglion in the wrist are the joint capsule on the radial aspect of the dorsal and volar sides of the wrist and the flexor tendon sheath in the midline of the finger at its proximal flexion crease.

■ Clinical Manifestations

The typical patient with a ganglion is a woman between 20 and 50 years old who complains of a rapidly developing painless lump. Sometimes the lump grows so quickly that it happens overnight. Depending on the location of the ganglion, it may or may not be painful or limit function. For example, a dorsal wrist ganglion may cause pain by stretching the posterior interosseous nerve as it provides sensory innervation to the dorsal wrist capsule. In such a patient, grip strength may also be decreased secondary to pain. In a patient with a flexor tendon sheath ganglion, the patient may have pain with gripping objects, such as a steering wheel or book.

Sometimes a patient will mention that the cyst increases and decreases in size. This is an important symptom to note because it makes the diagnosis of ganglion much more certain and neoplasm less likely, because neoplasms do not generally wax and wane in size in that manner. In some patients, pain may be the first symptom, and the lump may not develop until weeks or months later.

Physical Examination

On physical examination, the skin overlying the ganglion is found to be freely mobile, but the ganglion is generally firm and fixed to the deep tissue. By darkening the room, the examiner may shine a penlight and transilluminate the fluid-filled pseudocyst. Depending on the location, the ganglion may or may not be tender.

■ Diagnostic Evaluation

Needle aspiration of the ganglion yields a characteristic clear, thick fluid, which confirms the diagnosis. Anterior wrist ganglions are not aspirated out of concern for perforating the radial artery.

■ Treatment

In approximately 50% of patients, simple aspiration is both diagnostic and curative. The decision to remove a ganglion via surgery is a clinical one based on symptoms. Common surgical indications include pain, cosmetic deformity, and uncharacteristic-appearing fluid on aspiration. The important part of the surgical procedure is not removing the mass, but rather taking care to remove the entirety of the joint capsule or tendon sheath producing the fluid. Five percent of ganglions recur after operation as a result of incomplete excision. Recurrences are treated with repeat surgery, in which wider margins of the capsule or tendon sheath are taken.

Kienbock's Disease

Avascular necrosis and collapse of the lunate leading to carpal collapse was first described in 1910 by Kienbock. Ultimately, this disease progresses to generalized wrist arthrosis. It is not clear if the lunate fracture is the result or cause of the osteonecrosis. In any case, repetitive microtrauma is believed to play a prominent role in the evolution of the disease process.

■ Clinical Manifestations

The typical patient is a young adult who presents with a complaint of aching and stiffness in the wrist. On physical examination, the lunate is found to be tender. Grip strength is generally decreased. Range of motion may become restricted as the disease progresses.

■ Diagnostic Evaluation

Plain film radiographs should be obtained. The earliest changes in Kienbock's disease that are seen on radiograph include increased density of the lunate bone. Next, compressive forces generated between the distal capitate and proximal radius lead to collapse of the weakened lunate. This collapse leads to a flattened, sclerotic appearance on radiograph. Diffuse severe osteoarthritis in the intercarpal and radiocarpal bones develop after the lunate collapses.

Bone scan is helpful in the early diagnosis of Kienbock's disease. Before the increased density of the lunate is seen on radiograph, a bone scan will reveal increased uptake in the lunate.

■ Treatment

Kienbock's disease does not carry a good prognosis. Before fragmentation of the lunate, treatment is with surgery designed to decrease the load on the lunate. Later in the disease, salvage surgery in the form of a carpectomy or wrist arthrodesis may be necessary.

Distal Radius Fracture

Distal radius fractures are the most common encountered in orthopedic practices. In 1814 Colles described a transverse fracture of the distal radius with dorsal displacement of the distal fragment. This fracture continues to bear his name.

■ Clinical Manifestations

The typical patient is an elderly woman who reports a history of a fall onto an outstretched arm followed by pain and swelling. On physical examination, the classic clinical finding is the "dinner-fork

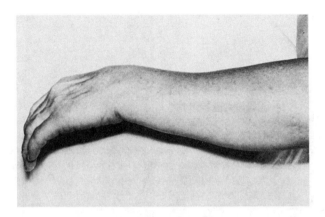

Figure 4-5 • Colles' fracture exhibiting the "dinner fork deformity" of the forearm and wrist. (Reproduced with permission from Duckworth, T. *Lecture Notes on Orthopaedics and Fractures,* third edition. Figure 16.2, p. 116. Blackwell Publishing, 1995).

deformity," in which there is a prominent bump on the dorsal wrist and a depression on the ventral side (Figure 4-5). The wrist is tender, and there is decreased range of motion.

■ Diagnostic Evaluation

Plain film radiographs, including anteroposterior (AP) and lateral views of the wrist, should be obtained (Figure 4-6 A and B). Computed tomography (CT) to better evaluate the bony defect may also be useful. Magnetic resonance imaging (MRI) may be helpful to evaluate for associated soft tissue injury.

■ Treatment

An attempt for closed reduction should be performed on any distal radius fracture. If it is possible to reduce the fracture temporarily, then external fixation with or without pins or screws, supplemental bone graft, or bone graft substitutes is performed. If a satisfactory reduction of the fracture cannot be accomplished via closed means, an open reduction with internal fixation may be necessary. Early mobilization following surgery is critical to maximize recovery.

Scaphoid Fracture

Almost 75% of all carpal fractures are scaphoid fractures. They are usually not seen in children or elderly patients. The scaphoid bone lies obliquely across the two rows of carpal bones in the

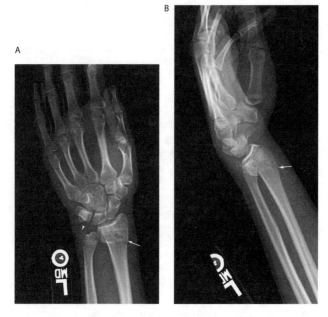

Figure 4-6 • Colles' fracture: (A) AP view and (B) lateral view. There is a fracture of the distal radius with mild dorsal angulation of the distal fragment. (Courtesy of Cedars-Sinai Medical Center, Los Angeles, California).

loading line between the thumb and forearm. The vascular supply of the scaphoid is strongest in the distal scaphoid and diminishes more proximally. This explains why 30% of midscaphoid fractures and more than 60% of proximal scaphoid fractures result in avascular necrosis.

■ Clinical Manifestations

The typical patient reports a history of a fall onto an outstretched arm. On physical examination, the classic finding is tenderness in the anatomic snuff box. The patient may also report pain with wrist extension. Grip strength may be diminished secondary to pain.

■ Diagnostic Evaluation

Plain film radiographs, including AP, lateral, and posteroanterior (PA) with ulnar deviation views, should be obtained (Figure 4-7). CT scan may be useful to better define the bony defect. MRI may be useful to better define the vascularity and surrounding soft tissue.

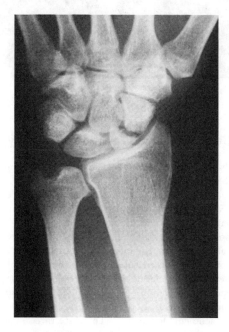

Figure 4-7 • Fracture of the scaphoid, avascular necrosis. (Reproduced with permission from Duckworth, T. *Lecture Notes on Orthopaedics and Fractures,* third edition. Figure 16.4, p. 120. Blackwell Publishing, 1995).

■ Treatment

If a patient has clinical symptoms but no radiographic evidence of fracture, a thumb spica may be used for two weeks, and then the patient may be reexamined. If a scaphoid tubercle fracture is present, it may be treated similar to a wrist sprain with only a bandage and early movement. Nondisplaced fractures are treated with strict immobilization. If the fracture is displaced, open reduction and internal fixation is necessary. Recently, bone grafts for proximal third fractures or avascular nonunions have been used with increasing frequency.

5 Thoracolumbar Spine

High-Yield Surgical and Functional Anatomy

The lumbar spine is more mobile than the thoracic spine and less mobile than the cervical spine. There are five lumbar vertebrae. The vertebral body is a large, box-shaped bone that serves the weight-bearing function of the vertebrae. The posterior elements of the vertebrae consist of the laminae, the articular processes, and the spinous processes. The inferior articular processes of one vertebra articulate with the inferior adjacent vertebra's superior articular processes. This articulation forms the zygapophyseal (Z) joints. The Z-joints are facet joints and prevent anterior-posterior displacement and rotation of the vertebrae upon one another. The spinous, transverse, and mamillary processes of the vertebrae provide attachments for muscles. There are three basic surgical approaches to the lumbar spine: posterior, anterior, and anterolateral.

■ Posterior Approach

The posterior approach to the lumbar spine is the most common and is used for excision of herniated discs, fusion surgery, and other pathologies. The spinous processes are easily palpated superficial structures. A convenient landmark is the superior aspect of the iliac crests, which denotes the L4-5 interspace. The superficial paraspinal muscles consist of the erector spinae, which are a group of vertically oriented muscles. The deeper paraspinal muscles run in an oblique pattern and include the multifidus and rotator muscles. At each lumbar level, the segmental lumbar vessels branch from the aorta and wrap around the waist of the vertebral body.

The spinal cord ends in the conus medullaris at approximately the L1 vertebral level. Nerve roots exit via the intervertebral foraminae of the superior body. For example, the L4 nerve root will exit between the L4 vertebrae and L5 vertebrae.

■ Anterior Approach

The anterior approach is useful for fusion surgery and other pathologies. The rectus abdominal muscles are found in the rectus sheath. Beneath the rectus sheath, several vital structures must be avoided. The dome of the bladder and other internal organs are present. The aorta runs along the left side of the vertebral column and bifurcates at the anterior surface of L4. The parasympathetic nerves in the presacral area run in a diffuse plexus surrounding the aorta. The ureters run inferior along the psoas muscle.

Adolescent Idiopathic Scoliosis

Scoliosis is a three-dimensional disorder of the spine. Approximately 80% of scoliosis is idiopathic. The prevalence of adolescent idiopathic scoliosis is 2% to 3%, and approximately 90% occurs in girls. Idiopathic scoliosis is defined radiographically as a Cobb angle of 10 degrees or greater with rotation. The Cobb angle is measured using posteroanterior (PA) films. First, a line is drawn across both the top of the superior end vertebra and the bottom of the inferior end vertebra. Another set of lines is drawn at 90-degree angles to the end vertebral lines. The intersection of these two lines is called the Cobb angle.

■ Clinical Manifestations

The typical patient is a girl between 10 and 17 years of age who may or may not give a history of her parents telling her she has an abnormal spinal curvature.

Physical Examination

Screening for scoliosis is done during routine checkups with primary care physicians. The patient is instructed to bend forward and trunk rotation is observed. If scoliosis is suspected, radiographs are obtained. A full neurologic examination should also be performed.

■ Diagnostic Evaluation

Plain film radiographs, including a PA of the full spine, should be obtained and the Cobb angle should be determined. Patients with abnormal curvatures (left thoracic curves), patients with spinal pain out of proportion to deformity, and patients with rapid curve progression documented by serial radiographs merit further investigation with magnetic resonance imaging (MRI). In addition, a patient with scoliosis and an abnormal neurologic examination should be further worked up with MRI.

■ Treatment

Treatment selection is guided primarily by likelihood of curve progression and functional impairments. Progression of the curve is most likely in young patients with large curvatures. Patients with curvatures less than 20 degrees should be watched with serial examinations and radiographs, but not necessarily treated. Patients with curves of between 20 and 40 degrees should be treated with full-time bracing. The bracing is continued until the patient achieves skeletal maturity. If the curve occurs at T8 or below, a plastic thoracolumbosacral orthosis (TLSO) may be used. For curves above T8, a cervicothoracolumbosacral orthosis (CTLSO) or Milwaukee brace is indicated.

Surgical intervention is typically reserved for patients with skeletal immaturity who have failed bracing treatment and have curves greater than 40 degrees, or in patients with curves greater than 50 degrees, especially if the patient has associated functional impairment.

When surgical intervention is pursued, the levels of instrumentation and fusion must be decided. Posterior spinal fusion and instrumentation with a multirod, hook, and screw system from a neutral vertebra to a stable vertebra below is a standard approach. The anterior approach has a higher rate of pseudoarthrosis, rod breakage, and incomplete correction. However, the anterior approach does reduce the number of levels that need to be fused. In general, potential complications include spinal cord or nerve root injury, infection, pseudoarthrosis, and instrumentation failure.

Low Back Pain

Low back pain (LBP) is a broad, common, and much debated subject. As much as 70% of the population will have back pain at some point in their life. Most acute cases of LBP (defined as back pain lasting less than 3 months) are believed to resolve spontaneously. When back pain becomes chronic (defined as lasting more than 3 months), there are three main identifiable causes. In approximately 39% of patients with chronic low back pain (CLBP), the cause is found to originate from an intervertebral disc. In approximately 15% of patients, the cause is found to originate from the sacroiliac joint. In approximately 15% of working-age patients, the cause of CLBP has been found to be the Z-joints. In approximately 40% of elderly patients, the cause of CLBP has been found to be the Z-joints.

■ Clinical Manifestations

The typical patient presents with a complaint of chronic axial LBP for longer than 3 months. There may or may not be a precipitating traumatic insult such as a back strain while lifting a heavy object or twisting suddenly. In many patients, the onset is insidious. Patients may complain of pain in their hips and/or knees. This pain is dull and vague *in contrast* to radicular pain, which is more typically radiating, electric, and bandlike.

All patients with LBP should be screened for red flag symptoms, which include any night sweats; weight loss; hematuria; urinary retention, frequency, or hesitancy; cough; history of cancer; overseas travel; recent surgery; fever; or increased pain at rest. Patients who answer "yes" to any of these symptoms may have a more serious underlying condition such as cancer or infection, and this diagnosis should be pursued and ruled out first. Patients older than age 50 are also at increased risk for an underlying cancer.

Physical Examination

The physical examination is essentially unrevealing in a patient with uncomplicated chronic axial LBP. There may be pain with bending over. This may suggest a discogenic origination of the pain because forward flexion increases stress on the disc, but that point is debatable. There may be pain with extension and lateral rotation, which may suggest Z-joint pain because the maneuver stresses the Z-joints. However, again, this point is debatable and evidence to support this maneuver is inconclusive.

Tender trigger points may be found in the paraspinal muscles of the back, but these trigger points are more likely a result of the underlying cause of the CLBP, rather than the underlying cause itself. Nevertheless, they may exacerbate the patient's morbidity. The Fabere's or Patrick's test is used to identify patients with sacroiliac joint disease. In this test, the patient's hip is flexed, abducted, and externally rotated into a figure-four position. Pressure is then applied by the examiner onto the patient's bent knee and iliac bone on the opposite side of the pelvis (Figure 5-1). When this maneuver elicits pain in the patient, the test is positive. However, the reliability of this test is also unproven.

■ Diagnostic Evaluation

Plain film radiographs, including anteroposterior (AP) and lateral views, may be obtained, but they have not actually been found to add diagnostic value to the workup of uncomplicated CLBP in a younger patient. In patients older than age 50, plain film radiographs are additionally useful to help rule out an underlying cancer. MRI is another potential diagnostic imaging aid. However, although MRI may help rule out more serious underlying problems such as cancer and may suggest a discogenic cause if a high-intensity zone is found, the gold standard of diagnosis for CLBP remains diagnostic injections.

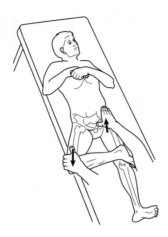

Figure 5-1 • Patrick's or Fabere's test. The hip is flexed, abducted, and externally rotated. (Reproduced with permission from Gross, J. *Musculoskeletal Examination*, second edition. Figure 6.66, p. 137. Blackwell Publishing, 2002).

Discogenic Pain

In order to diagnose discogenic CLBP, a provocative discogram with postdiscogram computed tomography (CT) evaluation needs to be obtained. In this test, dye is injected into the disc via a percutaneous needle. When this increased pressure from the dye reproduces the patient's typical pain, it is a positive test. On posttest CT examination, if there is a tear in the disc, then the dye is seen to extravasate from the nucleus pulposus into the annulus fibrosus.

Annulus Fibrosus Fissure

There are five potential grades of fissuring in the annulus fibrosus (Table 5-1). The sensory nerve fibers that are painful in the disc are found in the outer third of the annulus. Therefore, patients with positive provocative discography are typically found to have a grade III or greater annulus fissure.

Z-Joint Pain

In order to diagnose Z-joint pain, controlled diagnostic blocks of the dorsal branches of the medial rami innervating the painful joints is performed. This, too, is done percutaneously under fluoroscopic guidance. The Z-joint may also be blocked with controlled intra-articular injections under fluoroscopic guidance.

Sacroiliac Joint Pain

Because the anatomy of the nerve innervation of the sacroiliac is variable and has not been reliably delineated, the innervating nerves

Grade	Fissure
TABLE 5-1	Grades of Annulus Fibrosus Fissure
0	No fissure
I	Penetrates the inner third of the annulus
II	Penetrates the middle third of the annulus
III	Penetrates the outer third of the annulus
IV	Penetrates circumferentially around the rim of the annulus

cannot be reliably blocked. Instead, sacroiliac joint pain must be diagnosed using injections of controlled intra-articular local anesthetic blocks under fluoroscopic guidance.

■ Treatment

Acute LBP is treated with rest, nonsteroidal anti-inflammatory drugs (NSAIDs), stretching, heat, physical therapy, trigger point injections, tender point injections, or no treatment. Approximately 10% of patients with acute LBP will continue to have symptoms for longer than 3 months and are thus diagnosed with chronic low back pain. CLBP is much less likely to resolve on its own. When controlled diagnostic blocks of the dorsal medial rami determine that the underlying cause is Z-joint disease, radiofrequency neurotomy of the dorsal rami may be performed. This procedure essentially cuts the nerves innervating the painful joint(s). Without a nerve supply, the joint(s) no longer transmit(s) pain. The nerves may regenerate slowly over time, however, and the procedure may need to be periodically repeated.

When the underlying cause of CLBP is investigated with provocative discography and found to be the intervertebral disc (discogenic LBP), several choices for treatment are available. Conservative care consists primarily of physical therapy, heat, and NSAIDs. If conservative care is not effective, another minimally invasive technique is intradiscal electrothermal (IDET) annuloplasty. IDET is a percutaneous procedure in which a catheter is introduced under fluoroscopic guidance into the annulus of the disc. The catheter is then heated in order to destroy the nerves and denature the collagen. Radiofrequency neurotomy is another percutaneous minimally invasive option designed to reduce the intradiscal pressure in order to take some of the pressure off the injured annulus. When surgery is considered, preferred surgical options for discogenic CLBP include anterior lumbar interbody fusion and posterior lumbar interbody fusion. Posterolateral fusion appears to be less efficacious when compared with anterior or posterior interbody fusion methods.

Lumbosacral Radiculopathy

Lumbosacral radiculopathy occurs in roughly 2% of the population, making it relatively uncommon when compared with LBP. Nevertheless, lumbosacral radiculopathy is a source of significant morbidity in the general population. Risk factors for lumbosacral radiculopathy include male gender, job or activities involving twisting and/or heavy lifting, lower income, and tobacco intake.

Lumbosacral radiculopathy is a neurologic disorder resulting from compression or ischemia of the involved neurons. The compression may be a result of disc bulge, protrusion, extrusion, or sequestration, osteophytes from the disc or Z-joint, buckled ligamentum flavum, cyst, or tumor. The result of the compression is a block in the conduction of the involved spinal nerve or its roots. Radiculopathy, in its purest sense, is not a source of pain. Radiculopathy is a state of neurologic loss in which numbness or weakness results. However, radicular pain is caused by irritation of a spinal nerve or its roots and is often associated with radiculopathy. Therefore, radiculopathy and radicular pain are often discussed together.

■ Clinical Manifestations

The typical patient is an active male with a complaint of numbness, burning, and/or weakness radiating in a bandlike fashion down the thigh and leg. In a patient with spinal stenosis and radiculopathy, symptoms will often be alleviated with trunk flexion. These patients classically describe improvement in symptoms when grocery shopping because they are leaning forward on the grocery cart. In patients with a disc herniation, however, leaning forward typically exacerbates the symptoms and leaning backward alleviates the symptoms. The distribution of symptoms depends on the level of nerve root involvement. Figures 5-2 through 5-6 depict a summary of the segmental involvement and the tests to perform for each level.

It is important to ask patients about changes in bowel or bladder habits and previously listed red flag symptoms (see section on low back pain) in order to rule out more serious underlying conditions. Changes in bowel or bladder habits should prompt concern for conus medullaris or cauda equine syndrome. Patients should also be asked about progression of neurologic symptoms because this may indicate a surgical emergency. Table 5-2 lists the symptoms, weakness, and reflexes associated with different levels of radiculopathy.

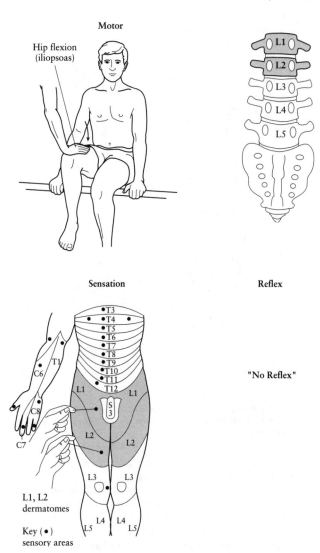

Figure 5-2 • The L1 and L2 root levels. (Reproduced with permission from Gross, J. *Musculoskeletal Examination,* second edition. Figure 6.48, p. 124. Blackwell Publishing, 2002).

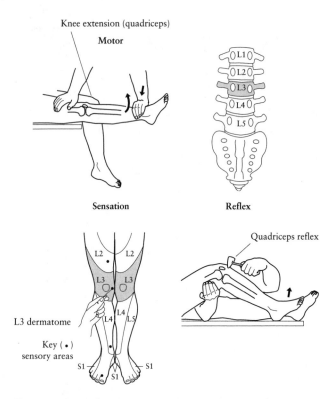

Figure 5-3 • The L3 root levels. (Reproduced with permission from Gross, J. *Musculoskeletal Examination*, second edition. Figure 6.49, p. 125. Blackwell Publishing, 2002).

Physical Examination

Straight-leg testing should be performed and is most sensitive for L5 and S1 radiculopathies. In this maneuver, the patient may be asked to sit down and lean forward with chin tucked down. The leg is then brought up and, if symptoms are reproduced, the test is positive. Another straight-leg test is to have the patient lie supine and passively flex the hip of one extended lower extremity at a time. At 35 to 70 degrees of extended leg elevation, the nerves are maximally stretched. After 70 degrees, the sciatic nerve in particular is deformed first distal to the neural foramen. Therefore, radicular symptoms reproduced with elevation past 70 degrees are unlikely to be caused by a disc herniation.

When the femoral nerve (L2-4) is suspected to be involved, a reverse straight-leg raise may be performed. In this maneuver, the

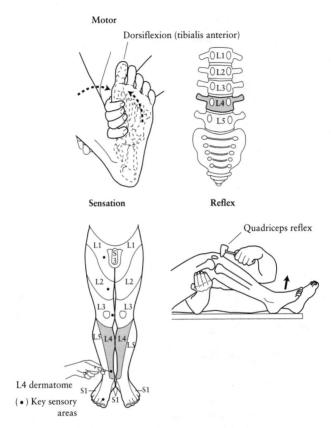

Motor

Dorsiflexion (tibialis anterior)

Sensation

Reflex

Quadriceps reflex

L4 dermatome

(•) Key sensory areas

Figure 5-4 • The L4 root level. (Reproduced with permission from Gross, J. *Musculoskeletal Examination,* second edition. Figure 6.50, p. 126. Blackwell Publishing, 2002).

patient is placed in the prone position and the lower extremity is put into hip extension and knee flexion. This maneuver evaluates the femoral nerve because of the anterior location of the nerve. If symptoms are reproduced, the test is positive.

The associated dermatomal distribution in a patient with a radiculopathy may reveal numbness or dysesthesia (see Table 5-2, p. 68). In a patient with an L5 radiculopathy, a Trendelenburg gait may be evident. During gait, the gluteus medius contracts to prevent the hip from dropping. The gluteus medius is innervated by L5, and so in a patient with an L5 radiculopathy, the gluteus medius may be weak and, during Trendelenburg gait, the patient's hip will slide toward the side of the lesion. See Figures 5-2 to 5-6 for an

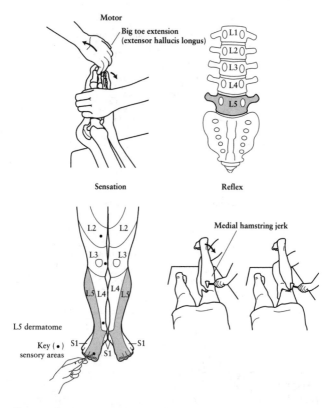

Figure 5-5 • The L5 root level. (Reproduced with permission from Gross, J. *Musculoskeletal Examination,* second edition. Figure 6.51, p. 128. Blackwell Publishing, 2002).

illustration of some of the important motor, sensory, and reflex testing for the respective nerve root segment involvement.

■ Diagnostic Evaluation

The natural history of radiculopathy is favorable in the acute phase. Therefore, in the first month, imaging may not be necessary. After 1 month, plain film radiographs and MRI should be obtained. It is critical to correlate clinical findings with MRI findings, because 37% of asymptomatic people may have evidence of disc abnormalities. When symptoms, straight-leg raising, and MRI are correlated, a disc herniation is found at surgery 95% of the time.

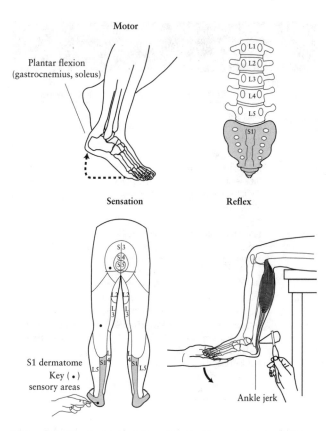

Figure 5-6 • The S1 root level. (Reproduced with permission from Gross, J. *Musculoskeletal Examination,* second edition. Figure 6.52, p. 129. Blackwell Publishing, 2002).

■ Treatment

Conservative care is the mainstay of initial treatment. Conservative management includes rest, a structured physical therapy program including stretching and strengthening exercises, NSAIDs, and heat. Epidural steroid and anesthetic injections delivered under fluoroscopic guidance are also very effective in the treatment of lumbosacral radiculopathy. The steroid and anesthetic injectate may be given via a caudal, interlaminar, or transforaminal route. Another minimally invasive option is percutaneous radiofrequency neurotomy.

For patients with a herniated disc, open discectomy is the gold standard surgical option. By surgically excising the displaced disc,

■ TABLE 5-2 Distribution of Sensory and Muscle Involvement for Different Neurologic Levels in Lumbosacral Radiculopathy

Neurologic Level	Sensory Distribution	Weakness	Reflex Involved
L3	Groin or medial aspect of the thigh; symptoms usually do not extend below the knee.		
L4	Anterior thigh, crossing the knee and entering the anteromedial leg, including the medial malleolus	Hip adductors and quadriceps (knee extensor)	Patellar reflex may be diminished or absent.
L5	Lateral thigh into the dorsum of the foot and the big toe	Extensor hallucis longus (classic muscle to test for L5), gluteus medius (hip abductor), and extensor digitorum longus and brevis	Trendelenburg gait may be evident.
S1	Posterior buttock, along the posterior thigh, into the lateral malleolus and foot, including the web space between the fourth and fifth toes	Plantarflexion	Achilles reflex may be diminished or absent.

the source of pressure and inflammation is removed. Other surgical procedures depend on the underlying pathology being treated. Patients with spinal stenosis may be treated with decompression surgeries such as laminectomy, hemilaminectomy, or laminotomy. When removing the lamina, care should be taken to preserve the pars interarticularis if possible in order to conserve stability.

Dysplastic and Isthmic Spondylolisthesis

Displacement of one vertebra anterior to the adjacent inferior vertebra is termed spondylolisthesis. Posterior displacement may also occur. Two types of spondylolisthesis include dysplastic and isthmic. Type I is congenital or dysplastic spondylolisthesis. Type II is isthmic or spondylitic spondylolisthesis. In type II spondylolisthesis, there is a defect in the pars interarticularis allowing the slippage.

■ Clinical Manifestations

The typical patient with type I spondylolisthesis is a female who participates in gymnastics (in which repetitive hyperextension is common) and who may complain of paresthesias in the involved segmental nerve distribution. For example, a patient with an L5 spondylolisthesis and impingement of the L5 nerve root may have paresthesias along the L5 nerve root distribution (see radiculopathy section for details). If not treated, symptoms may be progressive and lead to cauda equina syndrome.

The typical patient with type II spondylolisthesis is less likely to have neurologic involvement. Most patients with this defect are asymptomatic, and the finding is incidental on a radiograph taken for another reason. The slippage may progress with time. Rarely, type II spondylolisthesis is associated with low back pain.

Physical Examination

In a patient with paresthesias or radicular symptoms, the physical examination is consistent with that under the radiculopathy section. This is most applicable to type I spondylolisthesis, in which neurologic manifestations are common.

■ Diagnostic Evaluation

Plain film radiographs, including PA, lateral, and oblique views, are used to diagnose and monitor spondylolisthesis (Figure 5-7). CT and MRI are also useful. When spondylolisthesis is suspected as the cause of low back pain, a selective nerve block is useful in establishing the diagnosis.

■ Treatment

Children with symptomatic type I spondylolisthesis often require surgical intervention. Surgery may include decompression and stabilization or stabilization alone. Pedicle fixation is required for healthy adolescents and type I spondylolisthesis. In adults with symptomatic type I spondylolisthesis, conservative therapy may be attempted first. Conservative care includes a structured physical therapy program including stretching and strengthening exercises. If conservative care fails, surgery may be indicated.

Most patients with type II spondylolisthesis are asymptomatic and require no treatment. If a type II spondylolisthesis is discovered in children or adolescents, yearly serial radiographs should be obtained to monitor the slippage. Slips greater than 50% may be unstable and require surgery. Patients with type II spondylolisthesis and low back pain are often treated initially with physical therapy. Rarely, surgery may be indicated with pars interarticularis repair and early postoperative mobilization.

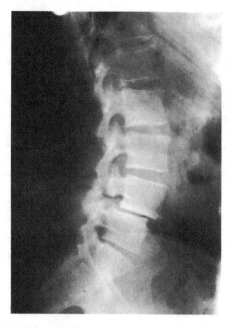

Figure 5-7 • Spondylolisthesis. (Reproduced with permission from Duckworth, T. *Lecture Notes on Orthopaedics and Fractures,* third edition. Figure 29.10, p. 229. Blackwell Publishing, 1995).

Osteoporotic Vertebral Compression Fracture

Vertebral compression fractures occur in 153 per 100,000 females and 81 per 100,000 males. Osteoporosis is a major risk factor for vertebral compression fractures. Of the 700,000 patients every year with vertebral compression fractures in the United States alone, 33% are symptomatic and require treatment, accounting for more than $1.5 billion in annual costs.

The typical pattern of vertebral compression fracture is wedge-shaped with gross collapse of the anterior portion of the vertebral body. A combination of spinal flexion and axial compression produces significant stresses on the anterior portion of the bone. In weakened osteoporotic bone, minimal flexion and/or axial loading may result in a compression fracture.

■ Clinical Manifestations

The typical patient with an osteoporotic compression fracture is a white or Asian woman older than age 65 who is asymptomatic. In this patient, the fracture is an asymptomatic finding on a radiograph taken for another reason. Other asymptomatic patients may only complain of height loss. Any patient with greater than 2 inches of height loss should be evaluated for a vertebral compression fracture. However, in the 33% of patients with symptomatic osteoporotic vertebral compression fractures, the typical patient is also a white or Asian woman who presents with a complaint of acute onset of axial pain following a low-exertion activity such as standing from a seated position, opening a window, or coughing. The pain is typically focal, but rarely the pain may wrap around the trunk of the body in a dermatomal distribution. Bowel or bladder changes are not characteristic of the diagnosis and, if present, warrant investigation into an alternate diagnosis.

Physical Examination

A normal-proportioned individual will stand with the fingertips hanging at midthigh. In a patient with fingertips extending to the lower thigh or knee, spinal shortening and compression fractures should be considered. During palpation of the patient's spine, tenderness will be elicited over the involved segments. In addition, asking the patient to bend over will typically exacerbate the pain.

■ Diagnostic Evaluation

Plain film radiographs, including PA and lateral views, should be obtained. The entire spine should be imaged because multiple fractures exist in as many as 20% of patients. It is essential to ascertain whether there is a laminar fracture, increased interpedicular space, or involvement of the posterior cortex because these findings may affect management. If vertebroplasty or kyphoplasty is considered, CT and/or MRI may be obtained to further evaluate for a defect in the posterior vertebral cortex. If metastatic disease is suspected, nuclear bone scanning should be obtained.

■ Treatment

When considering the initial intervention, the guiding characteristics are severity of pain, integrity of the posterior cortex, and percentage of vertebral collapse. If the posterior cortex is intact and the patient has severe pain and/or greater than 40% vertebral body collapse, vertebroplasty or kyphoplasty should be considered. Vertebroplasty is a percutaneous procedure in which a needle is inserted into the vertebral body and polymethylmethacrylate (PMMA) is injected under fluoroscopic guidance. Kyphoplasty is a newer procedure in which an inflatable bone tamp is inserted percutaneously under fluoroscopic guidance into the vertebral body and inflated. PMMA is then injected under low pressure into the cavity created by the inflatable bone tamp. The bone tamp is then deflated and removed. In this way, height is restored to the vertebral body. Contraindications to both procedures include a defect in the posterior cortex of the vertebral body.

In patients with less severe symptoms, less than 40% of collapse, or posterior cortex defect, conservative care is used. Conservative management includes physical therapy, heat, massage, NSAIDs, acetaminophen, bracing, and bed rest in order to provide symptomatic relief.

High-Yield Surgical and Functional Anatomy

The hip joint functions to connect the lower limb to the vertebral column. The hip joint is generally very stable. It is a large ball-and-socket-type joint. The primary hip flexor is the iliopsoas. The large iliopsoas muscle arises from the T12-L5, the iliac crest, iliac fossa, and sacrum and attaches onto the lesser trochanter. It is innervated by the ventral lumbar rami and the femoral nerve (L1,2,3). The primary hip extensor is the gluteus maximus, which is innervated by the inferior gluteal nerve (L5, S1,2). The primary hip abductor is the gluteus medius, which is innervated by the superior gluteal nerve (L5, S1). The gluteus minimus also abducts the hip and is also innervated by the superior gluteal nerve. The primary hip adductor is the adductor longus muscle, which is innervated by the obturator nerve (L2,3,4).

The primary ligaments of the hip are the capsular Y ligament, which is a strong stabilizer of the hip, and the intra-articular ligamentum teres. The typical surgical approaches to the hip include the anterior, anterolateral, and posterior approaches. The typical surgical approaches to the femur are lateral, posterolateral, anterolateral, and anteromedial.

■ Anterior Approach

The anterior surgical approach to the hip is used for open reduction of congenital dislocations, total hip replacement, hemiarthroplasty, and other pathologies. Superficial landmarks include the anterior superior iliac spine and the iliac crest. The sartorius muscle acts across two joints and is the most superficial muscle in the anterior thigh. It arises from the anterior superior iliac spine and inserts into the superior part of the medial surface of the tibia at the pes anserinus (a site that may become inflamed and cause pain). The sartorius flexes, abducts, and externally rotates the hip.

The femoral triangle consists of (from lateral to medial) the femoral nerve, femoral artery, the femoral vein, and lymphatics (remembered by the mnemonic: NAVEL–E is for empty space). The triangle also contains the lateral femoral cutaneous nerve and the femoral branch of the genitofemoral nerve. The triangle is bounded superiorly by the inguinal ligament, laterally by the sartorius muscle, and medially by the adductor longus muscle.

The femoral artery is a continuation of the external iliac artery. The femoral artery divides into the profunda femoris artery on the lateral side and the superficial femoral artery. The profunda femoris artery branches into the medial and lateral circumflex arteries that provide blood supply to the femoral neck.

The lateral femoral cutaneous nerve is not a branch of the femoral nerve. It is actually a direct branch from the lumbar plexus (L2,3). Injury to the lateral femoral cutaneous nerve may result in a painful neuroma and/or diminished sensation.

The quadriceps consists of the rectus femoris, vastus lateralis, vastus medialis, and vastus intermedius. These four muscles are innervated by the femoral nerve (L2-4) and insert via the patellar ligament onto the patella. The quadriceps work to extend the knee. The rectus femoris muscle also assists the iliopsoas in flexing the hip.

■ Posterior Approach

The posterior surgical approach to the hip is used for total hip replacement, hemiarthroplasty, open reduction and internal fixation of posterior acetabular fractures, and other pathologies. The greater trochanter is the primary superficial landmark. The sciatic nerve is formed by the posterior divisions of the ventral rami of L5 and S1,2. It is the largest nerve in the body and exits just below the piriformis muscle in the posterior approach to the hip. The sciatic nerve does not typically supply any structures in the gluteal region, and it divides halfway down the thigh to form the common peroneal and tibial nerves.

Developmental Dysplasia of the Hip

Developmental dysplasia of the hip (DDH) is the term used to describe a spectrum of disorders affecting the relationship between the proximal femur and acetabulum, resulting in hips that are subluxatable or dislocatable. Early diagnosis in infancy is critical because treatment is highly effective, and failure to treat may result in significant long-term morbidity.

Several variable factors interact to contribute to the development of DDH. In general, increased joint laxity and decreased hip mobility predispose to DDH. Genetics and increased levels of progesterone and relaxin during the final weeks of pregnancy contribute to DDH by increasing joint laxity. Oligohydramnios, breech position with extended legs, and carrying infants in a restricted position with legs together and hips and knees extended (as is customary in some native North American societies) predispose to DDH by restricting hip movement.

Approximately 5 to 20 per 1000 live births have hip instability. Most of these resolve, and at 3 weeks only 1 to 2 per 1000 live births have persistent instability. Girls are affected seven times as often as boys.

■ Clinical Manifestations

Optimally, all cases should be diagnosed by clinical exam at birth. However, many cases are not diagnosed until after birth. In late presentations, parents may report difficulty putting on the patient's diapers because of limited hip abduction. With unilateral dislocation, the skin creases are asymmetrical and the affected leg is slightly shorter and externally rotated. Although late walking is not a feature of DDH, any child who has not begun walking by 18 months must be evaluated for possible DDH.

Physical Examination

Two physical examination tests are commonly used to diagnose DDH. The Ortolani test is used to evaluate an already dislocated hip. It is performed by flexing the hips to 90 degrees and gently abducting them. In normal hips there is smooth abduction to almost 90 degrees. In a congenitally dislocated hip there is a palpable low-frequency "clunk" as the femoral head slides back and reduces into the acetabulum.

The Barlow test is used to determine if a hip is dislocatable. The femur is flexed and adducted as posterior pressure is applied. In an unstable hip, the femur will be easily dislocated from the acetabulum and then reduced again.

■ Diagnostic Evaluation

All patients with signs of instability should be evaluated with ultrasonography (US). US is highly sensitive for DDH and allows direct imaging of the cartilaginous portions of the hip that cannot be visualized on plain radiography. Some physicians advocate using US as a screening test for all infants to evaluate for DDH. Computed tomography (CT) and/or magnetic resonance imaging (MRI) may be useful in complicated cases. If US is available, plain film radiography is generally not indicated.

■ Differential Diagnosis

- DDH
- Tumor
- Trauma
- Septic arthritis

- Transient synovitis
- Congenital coax vara
- Legg-Calvé-Perthes disease

■ Treatment

Patients with a positive Ortolani or Barlow test but negative ultrasound should be observed for 3 to 6 months. If the ultrasound is still negative at 6 months, no intervention is necessary. Patients with a positive ultrasound examination should be splinted for 6 weeks and then reexamined with ultrasound. If the ultrasound is still positive, the splint should be continued for another 3 months and the patient should be reexamined again with ultrasound.

Splinting for DDH is designed to hold the hips somewhat flexed and abducted. The most important aspects of splinting are that the hip be properly reduced before splinting, extreme positions be avoided, and the hips retain some movement within the splint. The Pavlik harness is the most common splinting apparatus, and when used correctly has been shown to be 95% effective. The most common cause of failure of the Pavlik harness is patient noncompliance. Therefore, patient education and close follow-up is imperative.

In patients who are older than 18 months, splinting is unlikely to be successful and an open operation may be indicated. Before operation, a period of traction (at times combined with psoas and adductor tenotomy) is used to help loosen the tissues and allow the femoral head to move inferiorly opposite the acetabulum.

In patients with unilateral dislocation who are older than 10 years, the risk of surgery may be greater than the benefit. These patients often present with a painless limp and are found on evaluation to have previously undiagnosed DDH. The risk of open reduction is that the force required to reduce the hip may damage the vascular supply of the femoral head. These patients will usually remain pain free until midlife, when they may require a total hip replacement.

In patients with bilateral dislocation, the deformity and abnormal gait is often less marked, and an operation may not be indicated unless the patient develops pain or the deformity is particularly severe.

■ Follow-up

Infants are followed until they are able to walk without assistance. While using the Pavlik harness, patients are followed closely to adjust the harness and to ensure that it is being used correctly.

■ **Complications**

Missing the diagnosis may lead to persistent low back pain, hyperlordosis of the lumbar spine, secondary osteoarthritis, and sexual dysfunction in women with bilateral DDH who cannot abduct their hips.

Complications of the Pavlik harness include femoral nerve palsies, brachial plexus palsies, skin maceration and breakdown in the groin fold, and popliteal fossa. The most serious potential complication of the Pavlik harness is aseptic necrosis of the femoral head from excessive tightening of the abduction strap.

Legg-Calvé-Perthes Disease

Legg-Calvé-Perthes disease (LCPD) is a childhood hip disorder resulting from avascular necrosis (AVN) of the proximal femoral head. The incidence of LCPD is approximately 1 in 10,000. Ten percent of cases are bilateral. At birth the femoral head receives its blood supply from the metaphyseal vessels, the lateral epiphyseal vessels, and the ligamentum teres vessels. The ligamentum teres vessels do not fully develop until 7 years of age. The metaphyseal vessels disappear by age 4. Therefore, between 4 and 7 years of age, the only significant blood supply to the proximal femoral head is from the lateral epiphyseal vessels. A single trauma, multiple smaller traumas, or infection may compromise these vessels and lead to ischemia.

■ **Clinical Manifestations**

The typical patient is a boy between the ages of 4 and 7 who presents complaining of an insidious onset of a limp. When pain occurs, it is usually only related to activity and is relieved by rest. The pain is often located in the anterior thigh, but it may occur in the hip, groin, or knee.

Physical Examination
On physical examination, the patient may have an antalgic gait with limited hip motion. A Trendelenburg gait may be present caused by pain in the gluteus medius (see section on lumbosacral radiculopathy for discussion on Trendelenburg gait). Passive range of motion is often painful and limited, especially with internal rotation and abduction. The patient will often have evidence of thigh, calf, and buttock atrophy secondary to inactivity from pain.

■ **Diagnostic Evaluation**

Plain radiography remains the modality of choice to investigate suspected LCPD (Figure 6-1). Staging of LCPD is based on

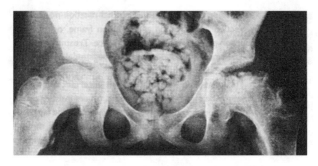

Figure 6-1 • Legg-Calvé-Perthes disease, showing fragmentation of the head. (Reproduced with permission from Duckworth, T. *Lecture Notes on Orthopaedics and Fractures,* third edition. Figure 30.2, p. 233. Blackwell Publishing, 1995).

■ TABLE 6-1 Salter-Thomson Classification and Caterall Staging		
Salter-Thomson Grouping	Caterall Stage	Plain Film Findings
A < 50% of head involved	I	No findings
	II	Sclerosis with or without cystic changes and preservation of femoral head
B > 50% of head involved	III	Loss of structural integrity of femoral head
	IV	Loss of structural integrity of acetabulum

anteroposterior (AP) and frog-leg views. Classically, the Caterall staging is used (Table 6-1).

Salter-Thomson classification simplified the staging system into groups A and B (see Table 6-1). Salter-Thomson group A includes Caterall stages I and II and indicates less than 50% of the femoral head involved. Group B includes stages III and IV and indicates greater than 50% of the femoral head involved.

CT scan allows early diagnosis of bone collapse, but the increased radiation exposure has decreased the utility of CT scanning for this disorder. MRI has the greatest sensitivity for LCPD, but bone marrow and joint effusion changes are nonspecific. The cost of MRI makes plain radiography a superior first choice.

■ **Treatment**

The goals of treatment are to prevent deformity, alter growth disturbances, and prevent the future premature development of degenerative joint disease. Sixty percent of children with LCPD do not require treatment. Children younger than 6 years of age have a better prognosis. Children younger than 4 years of age with less than 50% femoral head involvement (Salter-Thomson group A) generally do not require surgery. Older children with radiographic changes but excellent range of motion require close follow-up, but not necessarily treatment.

If the hip is irritable, the child should be placed in bed and skin traction ought to be applied to the affected leg in slight flexion and external rotation. Occasionally, surgical release of the contracted adductors is necessary. As the irritability subsides (usually after approximately 3 weeks), movement is encouraged. Once irritability has subsided, the primary goal of treatment is containment of the femur within the acetabulum. This goal is accomplished either via surgery or bracing. A brace, such as the Scottish Rite brace, internally rotates and abducts the hip, keeping the femoral head within the acetabulum while allowing full knee movement.

Surgical containment is often the preferred method because of superior results and a quicker return to normal social functioning. Surgical containment may be achieved via either a varus derotational osteotomy of the femur or an innominate osteotomy of the acetabulum. Following surgery, a plaster brace is used for approximately 2 months until the osteotomy has united.

■ Follow-up

Once symptoms have completely abated and radiography reveals healing, the child is permitted to resume full activity and return only as needed.

■ Complications

Failure to adequately treat LCPD may result in early-onset secondary osteoarthritis, possibly necessitating total hip replacement.

Transient Synovitis

Transient synovitis (TS) is the most common cause of acute hip pain in children ages 3 to 12 years. This self-limiting condition has an incidence of approximately 3%. Although the cause of TS remains elusive, a large percentage of children with TS have a recent history of an upper respiratory tract infection (URI), prompting suspicion of an underlying viral etiology.

■ Clinical Manifestations

The typical patient is a male who presents with unilateral hip or groin pain and/or a limp. The pain is sometimes experienced only in the anterior thigh, groin, or knee and may be severe enough to wake the child from sleep. Symptoms are usually intermittent and exacerbated by activity. In about half of all patients with TS, focused questioning will reveal a recent history of a URI, bronchitis, or otitis media. Children with TS rarely report a high fever, but they may have a mildly elevated temperature.

Physical Examination

On physical examination, there is guarded hip internal and external rotation. Passive range of motion, particularly through abduction and internal rotation, is painful. A sensitive test for TS is the "log roll." In this test, the patient is placed in the supine position, and the examiner gently rolls the patient's involved leg from external to internal rotation. Involuntary muscle guarding during this maneuver is considered a positive test.

■ Diagnostic Evaluation

Complete blood count (CBC), erythrocyte sedimentation rate (ESR), and X-ray examinations are all usually normal. The ESR is occasionally slightly elevated. X-ray may reveal an accentuated pericapsular shadow.

Ultrasound may show an effusion. Ultrasound may also be used to guide needle aspiration of the joint. Aspiration must be performed in all patients whenever the diagnosis of septic arthritis is considered. CT, MRI, and bone scan are not routinely indicated in the diagnostic workup of TS.

■ Differential Diagnosis

- Legg-Calvé-Perthe disease
- Slipped capital femoral epiphysis
- Septic arthritis
- Tumor
- Rheumatic arthralgias
- Juvenile chronic arthritis
- Lyme arthritis
- Avascular necrosis

■ Treatment

Initial treatment for patients with TS includes rest. Heat and massage may be used for symptom relief. If heat and massage fail to relieve symptoms, then nonsteroidal anti-inflammatory drugs (NSAIDs) may be used in the short term. As symptoms improve, the patient may begin to use crutches for ambulation. Full weight-bearing activities should be gradually resumed as symptoms abate. Most patients will have resolution of their symptoms within 1 week. However, in some patients symptoms may persist for months.

■ Complications

Complications are rare unless the child is allowed to resume activities before resolution of symptoms. When this happens, complications frequently include recurrent pain and inflammation. It is unclear whether TS places a child at risk for earlier development of degenerative joint disease.

Slipped Capital Femoral Epiphysis

Slipped capital femoral epiphysis (SCFE) is one of the most common adolescent hip disorders. In SCFE there is displacement of the capital femoral epiphysis from the metaphysis through the physeal plate, most frequently resulting in an aching sensation in the groin, thigh, and/or knee. Delay in diagnosis may result in long-term morbidity and early development of secondary osteoarthritis.

SCFE is a multifactorial disorder. During the pubertal growth spurt (when SCFE almost exclusively occurs), an imbalance between pituitary hormonal activity and increasing gonadal hormonal activity may weaken the physeal plate, making it unable to cope with the shearing stresses of increasing body weight and/or traumatic insult.

■ Clinical Manifestations

The typical patient is an overweight male boy in puberty who presents with a complaint of a limp and a vague aching sensation in the groin, thigh, or knee. Fifty percent of all patients recall a history of trauma. The left hip is involved more frequently than the right. The patient often reports a history of relapsing and remitting symptoms that are better with rest and exacerbated by activity. This intermittent symptom pattern reflects a series of minor, intermittent slips. These patients will often eventually experience an acute painful episode (the "acute on chronic" slip).

Physical Examination

On physical examination, the typical patient is obese with an affected leg that is 1 to 2 cm short and externally rotated. Patients will almost uniformly have an asymmetric out-toeing gait and limp. Patients typically have limitation of hip flexion, abduction, and internal rotation. The patient often will also increase external rotation during hip flexion. Following an acute severe slip, all passive and active movements of the hip are painful.

■ Diagnostic Evaluation

Radiographs, including AP, lateral, and frog-leg views, should be obtained. On the AP view, a line drawn along the superior border of the femoral neck should pass through a portion of the femoral head. Failure of the line to pass through the head (Trethowan's sign) is diagnostic of SCFE. The image of SCFE on radiograph has also been described as having an "ice cream falling off a cone" appearance.

CT and MRI are more sensitive for SCFE, but they are not indicated except rarely in early cases of suspected SCFE with negative radiographs. CT scans may also be helpful in delineating the exact direction and degree of displacement.

■ Treatment

Once the diagnosis of SCFE is made, the patient should be made non-weight-bearing, and treatment should be considered an emergency. Delay in treatment risks further slippage and potential compromise of the remaining intact blood supply to the epiphysis, potentially resulting in AVN. Further treatment depends on the degree of slippage. Most cases of SCFE have mild (less than 25%) or moderate (25% to 50%) slippage. For these patients, the preferred surgical intervention is internal fixation using either central percutaneous pin fixation with one or more cannulated screws or multiple smooth Kirschner wires. When performed properly, this procedure is very well tolerated.

In patients with severe slippage (more than 50%), the slip causes marked deformity and morbidity and, if untreated, will lead to early secondary osteoarthritis. Severe slips may be treated with no reduction and pinning (as in mild and moderate slips), closed reduction and pinning, or open reduction with or without osteotomy and pinning.

Postoperatively patients are given crutches and kept to light weight-bearing for approximately 6 to 8 weeks. Once pain has resolved and a comfortable range of motion has been achieved, rapid advance to full weight-bearing may begin.

■ Follow-up

Each patient must be followed closely until the patient is pain free and radiographic examination reveals physeal closure.

■ Complications

AVN is the most serious potential complication and may occur as a result of vascular damage from a severe acute slip or from overly aggressive reduction of even a mild slip. Chondrolysis, or cartilage necrosis, is often associated with SCFE and may manifest as loss of range of motion, pain, limp, and/or joint contracture. The cause of this association is not fully appreciated but appears to be related to prolonged immobilization, pin penetration, and long duration of slips before treatment. Secondary osteoarthritis of the hip is also a potential complication from delaying treatment, not treating, or inadequately treating SCFE.

Osteoarthritis of the Hip

Osteoarthritis (OA) is the most common form of progressive joint disease worldwide. By the year 2020, approximately 60 million people in the United States alone are expected to be affected. OA is commonly seen in the elderly but may occur much earlier in certain patients. It is characterized by progressive cartilage degeneration and is particularly found in weight-bearing joints. The hip is one of the most commonly involved joints in OA.

In OA, repetitive microtrauma in the articular cartilage of the hip leads to a localized immune reaction and further damage. The initial stage is generally swelling of the cartilage caused by an increased synthesis of proteoglycans. As OA progresses, the joint surface thickness is eroded and the number of proteoglycans becomes reduced, leading to cartilage softening and exposing the subchondral bone. This prompts the development of bone cysts. Endochondral ossification is stimulated and osteophytes result. Synovial hypertrophy is common, and capsular fibrosis may account for joint stiffness.

Risk factors for hip OA include increased age, obesity, female, any condition predisposing to secondary OA (e.g., history of LCPD, SCFE, hemochromatosis, Wilson's disease, AVN, gout, Paget's disease, neuropathic disorders, hyperparathyroidism, rheumatoid arthritis, septic arthritis, hemophilia), mechanical stress, and/or joint trauma.

■ Clinical Manifestations

The typical patient is older than age 50 and presents with a complaint of pain in the groin that may refer to the knee. The pain typically occurs after periods of activity. As the disease progresses, the pain becomes more constant and at times will even disturb sleep. The patient will initially complain of stiffness at rest. However, as the disease progresses, the stiffness increases until putting on shoes and socks is difficult. Patients also often complain of limping because of the pain.

Physical Examination

On physical examination, patients may demonstrate an antalgic gait. The affected leg usually lies in external rotation and adduction, giving it the appearance of being shorter than the unaffected leg. Range of motion is often restricted secondary to pain. Hip internal rotation, abduction, and extension are affected first and with the most severity.

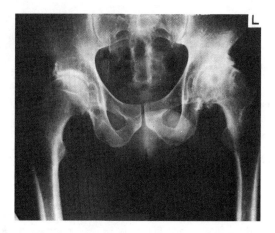

Figure 6-2 • X-ray appearance of osteoarthritic hip. (Reproduced with permission from Duckworth, T. *Lecture Notes on Orthopaedics and Fractures,* third edition. Figure 46.6, p. 361. Blackwell Publishing, 1995).

■ Diagnostic Evaluation

Plain radiographs, including AP and lateral views, are the most appropriate imaging modality to investigate OA. Initial X-ray will reveal decreased joint space, particularly in the superior weight-bearing region. Later in the disease, X-ray will show sub-articular sclerosis, cyst formation, and osteophytes (Figure 6-2). Importantly, the extent of OA changes found on X-ray *do not* necessarily correlate with clinical symptoms. Patients with severe osteoarthritic changes on X-ray may have few or no symptoms. Likewise, patients with severe, disabling symptoms may have minimal osteoarthritic changes on X-ray.

■ Differential Diagnosis

- Avascular necrosis
- Rheumatoid arthritis
- Lyme arthritis
- Septic arthritis
- Crystalline arthritis

■ Treatment

The decision to treat OA of the hip is based on symptoms and comorbidities, not radiographic findings.

Conservative Care

Conservative care focuses on protecting the joint, reducing symptoms, and restoring function. Reducing stressful activities, resting, weight reduction (when appropriate), using ambulatory aides (e.g., cane), heat, gentle range-of-motion exercises, nonimpact exercises (e.g., swimming), and muscle strengthening exercises are the cornerstone interventions for conservative care. Recently, glucosamine sulfate (1500 mg) and chondroitin sulfate (1200 mg) have attracted considerable attention in the literature. Preliminary studies indicate that taking the combination of the two nutraceuticals offers symptomatic relief from hip OA.

Surgical Intervention

When conservative care fails, surgical intervention should be considered. The decision to treat surgically is largely guided by the patient's comorbidities, expectations, and degree of symptoms. The most common surgery for hip OA is total hip replacement (see following section on total hip replacement). In addition, recent research has focused on two new procedures aimed at biologically healing and regenerating osteoarthritic cartilage. Autogenous osteochondral grafting (mosaicplasty) and autologous chondrocyte implantation (ACI) have been used with promising results for OA in the knee. These procedures are not currently used in the hip, but research is ongoing.

TOTAL HIP REPLACEMENT

A total hip replacement (THR) involves replacing the femoral head and acetabular surface. The attempt of a total joint replacement is to reproduce the physiologic joint.

Hemiarthroplasty involves replacing only the femoral head. The prosthesis used may be fixed with polymethylmethacrylate cement or without cement. Cement fixation offers the advantage of being the strongest fixation immediately after surgery. Patients with cement prostheses are weight-bearing as tolerated after surgery and have less pain after surgery. The most common complication of cement fixation is loosening of the prosthesis.

With cementless procedures, patients must remain toe-touch weight-bearing (i.e., may put only about 10% of their weight onto the affected limb) for approximately 6 weeks and are then progressed to weight-bearing as tolerated. Following a cementless procedure, patients also typically experience greater pain than after a cemented procedure. Cementless procedures have the advantage of a stronger overall fixation once the bony ingrowth has occurred. In general, cemented procedures are preferred in elderly patients and cementless procedures are preferred in younger patients.

Following a THR (assuming a posterior approach is used), hip precautions include no hip flexion past 90 degrees, no hip adduction beyond neutral, and no hip internal rotation past neutral. If an anterior approach is used for the hip replacement, these hip precautions are reverse such that there may be no extension past neutral, no adduction past midline, and no external rotation. Hip precautions are followed for 3 to 6 months.

In patients with cemented devices who are weight-bearing as tolerated on day number two, gait training with assistive devices and functional transferring training is initiated. Progressive range-of-motion and strengthening exercises are also begun and continued for approximately 1 month.

A serious potential complication of THR is thromboembolic disease, including deep venous thrombosis (DVT) and potentially fatal pulmonary embolus (PE). In fact, greater than 50% of patients who are not anticoagulated after THR develop a DVT. For this reason, patients are generally anticoagulated following a THR. Warfarin (keeping the International Normalized Ratio [INR] between 2 and 3) may be used. Low-molecular-weight heparin or subcutaneous heparin 5000 units twice a day may also be used. Some surgeons also use 325 mg aspirin twice a day. In patients who have contraindications to anticoagulation, intermittent pneumatic stockings or PlexiPulse boots may be used. Patients at high risk for DVT or PE who are not candidates for anticoagulation therapy may require inferior vena cava filter placement.

Other potential complications of a total hip replacement include failure of the prosthesis, infection, heterotopic bone ossification, acetabular wear, and leg length discrepancy. It is important to monitor and correct any leg length discrepancy with orthoses or heel lifts.

Rheumatoid Arthritis of the Hip

The hip joint is less frequently involved than other joints in rheumatoid arthritis (RA). However, when the hip is involved in RA, significant morbidity may result. In RA of the hip, the acetabulum may eventually be eroded to the point that the femoral head perforates its floor.

■ Clinical Manifestations

The patient is typically a female between the ages of 40 and 60 who presents with a history of RA in other joints and a new complaint of insidious onset of pain in the groin. As the disease advances, the patient may report difficulty getting in and out of bed, and even movements in bed may become painful. At times the slow progression of RA may be punctuated by acute, intense flares of hip and/or groin pain. Limp, although certainly common, may often be attributed to preexisting RA in the knee or foot.

Physical Examination

On physical examination, signs of RA are usually already present in other joints of the body. In the hip, wasting of the buttock and thigh may be noted. The patient may hold the involved limb in external rotation and fixed flexion. Both passive and active range of motion of the hip will be restricted and painful.

■ Diagnostic Evaluation

Blood work, including CBC, ESR, antinuclear antibody (ANA), and rheumatoid factor (RF), should be obtained. Plain radiographs of the hip joint may reveal varying degrees of osteopenia and loss of joint space. In contrast to the OA of the hip, in RA the loss of joint space is typically concentric. In the worst cases, and particularly in patients on corticosteroids, there may be gross bone destruction and the floor of the acetabulum may be perforated. Osteophytes are rare in RA.

■ Differential Diagnosis

- Avascular necrosis
- Osteoarthritis
- Lyme arthritis
- Septic arthritis
- Crystalline arthritis

■ Treatment

Treating the underlying systemic RA is central to treating RA of the hip. Systemic therapy, including glucocorticoids, methotrexate, etanercept, infliximab, and other disease-modifying antirheumatic drugs, is particularly useful. In addition, conservative care similar to the methods described previously in treating OA of the hip should be utilized. Intra-articular corticosteroid injections may also be helpful in hip RA. When surgery is indicated, THR remains the mainstay of treatment for both juvenile RA and adult RA (see subsection regarding THR in hip OA section).

Hip Dislocation

A severe force is required to cause a hip dislocation. Hip dislocations are classified according to the direction of dislocation. In posterior hip dislocation, the head of the femur is displaced posterior to the acetabulum while the thigh is flexed. Commonly, a posterior dislocation will result from a head-on automobile accident in which the knee is driven forcefully into the dashboard. Approximately 7% of posterior dislocations are accompanied by a femoral head or neck fracture.

In anterior dislocation, the femoral head generally remains lateral to the obturator externus muscle. This type of dislocation usually results when impact occurs at a time that the hip is extended and externally rotated.

Posterior dislocations account for as much as 85% to 90% of all hip dislocations. Anterior dislocations account for 10% to 18% of all hip dislocations.

■ Clinical Manifestations

Patients with hip dislocations almost universally present with a history of significant trauma. A classic presentation for a posterior hip dislocation is a head-on, high-speed motor vehicle accident. Patients will complain of pain and swelling.

Physical Examination

Significant clinical findings in posterior dislocations include shortening, adduction, and internal rotation of the extremity. In anterior hip dislocations, the hip is classically flexed, abducted, and externally rotated.

■ Diagnostic Evaluation

Plain film radiograph is the primary imaging modality and should include X-rays of the pelvis and entire femur to identify the most commonly associated injuries, which include fractures of the acetabulum, ipsilateral femoral head, neck and/or shaft, and pelvis.

■ Differential Diagnosis

- Hip dislocation
- Fracture of the acetabulum, ipsilateral femoral head, neck and/or shaft, and pelvis

■ Treatment

A posterior dislocation is treated with closed reduction by traction on the adducted and flexed hip. X-rays are obtained after reduction to confirm a concentric reduction. If the initial reduction is unsuccessful, then a closed reduction under general anesthesia with muscle paralysis should be attempted. A percutaneous Schanz pin at the subtrochanteric level may be used to manipulate the femur. If this is still unsuccessful in obtaining a concentric reduction, then a CT scan is obtained followed by open reduction. CT can also be used postoperatively to assess stability of the reduction.

A posterior dislocation associated with a femoral head fracture is treated with open reduction if closed reduction under general anesthesia fails to achieve concentric reduction. A posterior dislocation associated with a femoral neck fracture is always treated with open reduction and internal fixation of the fracture.

An anterior hip dislocation is treated with closed reduction by traction in line with the femur. Next, traction is used in hip extension and internal rotation.

■ Follow-up

AVN has been reported to occur as late as 2 years after initial injury. Therefore, after treatment it is important to maintain adequate follow-up during this time. Patients should be enrolled in a structured physical therapy program soon after surgical intervention, and they should be monitored periodically for any changes in their condition for at least 2 years.

■ Complications

Complications from posterior and anterior hip dislocations include infection, AVN of the femoral head, malunion, posttraumatic degenerative joint disease, and recurrent dislocation. Risk of AVN has been shown to be reduced if reduction of the dislocation is performed within 6 hours of injury. Sciatic nerve injury has been reported, occurring in up to 10% to 20% of patients with posterior hip dislocation.

Hip Fracture

Hip fractures include intertrochanteric and femoral neck fractures and are a source of serious morbidity and mortality (Figure 6-3). Most hip fractures are a result of low-energy impact and occur in the elderly population. In older patients, weakened bones from osteoporosis, arthritis, and deconditioning predispose the hip to fracture. Likewise, deconditioning, age-related neuromuscular decline in function, and vision changes may increase the likelihood for a fall.

Hip fractures in patients younger than 50 years of age are rare and are almost always the result of high-energy trauma such as from a high-speed motor vehicle accident. The incidence of hip fracture doubles during each decade that a person lives beyond 50 years of age. Women are twice as likely to be affected as men. The 1-year mortality rate following a hip fracture in older patients ranges from 14% to 36%, which is greater than for age-matched controls.

■ Clinical Manifestations

A typical history is an elderly man or woman who reports falling and subsequently having pain in the hip, groin, thigh, or knee.

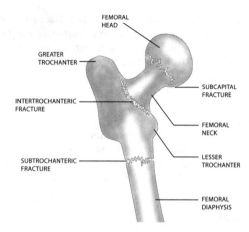

Figure 6-3 • Diagram of common points of femoral fracture. (Reproduced with permission from Uzelac, A. *Blueprints Radiology,* second edition. Figure 8-10. Blackwell Publishing, 2006).

The patient will report having trouble with weight-bearing, and motion at the hip joint may be difficult.

Physical Examination

On physical examination, in femoral neck fractures the involved extremity may be slightly shortened and externally rotated. In intertrochanteric fractures, the involved extremity may be shortened and internally rotated. Hip motion may be painful (except in some nondisplaced fractures).

■ Diagnostic Evaluation

Plain film radiographs, including AP of the pelvis, groin, and lateral views, are the imaging modality of first choice. In femoral neck fractures, the Garden classification is the most widely used system (Table 6-2). Higher Garden classifications have a higher association with the subsequent development of AVN.

Intertrochanteric fractures may reveal a disruption of the cortex or as a lucent fracture line (Figure 6-4). Intertrochanteric fractures may also be displaced and show an abnormality in the normal relationship of the femur. The Jensen classification may be used to characterize intertrochanteric fractures (Table 6-3).

Suspected hip fractures with normal radiographic findings may be further worked up using a combination of T1- and T2-weighted MRI images. One study found that 67% of patients seen in an emergency room with posttraumatic hip pain had normal X-rays and occult hip fracture revealed on MRI.

Garden Type	Findings	Treatment
I	Femoral head valgus impaction	Open reduction internal fixation
II	Complete, nondisplaced fracture	Open reduction internal fixation
III	Varus displacement of femoral head	Open or closed fixation versus total hip replacement
IV	Complete loss of fragment continuity	Open or closed fixation versus total hip replacement

TABLE 6-2 Garden Classification and Treatment

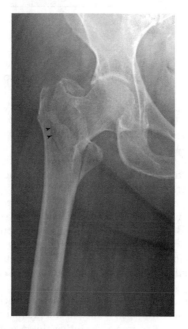

Figure 6-4 • Hip fracture. Intertrochanteric fracture in the right hip of an 83-year-old woman who fell after getting out of bed. (Courtesy of Cedars-Sinai Medical Center, Los Angeles, California).

■ Differential Diagnosis

- Femoral neck fracture
- Intertrochanteric fracture
- Subtrochanteric fracture
- Femoral shaft fracture
- Hip dislocation
- Acetabulum fracture

■ TABLE 6-3 Jensen Classification of Intertrochanteric Fractures		
Type	Findings	Stability
I	Nondisplaced two-fragment fracture	Stable
II	Displaced two-fragment fracture	Stable
III	Three-fragment fracture without posterolateral support	Unstable
IV	Three-fragment fracture without medial support	Unstable
V	Four-fragment fracture without posterolateral and medial support	Unstable

■ Treatment

Garden type I and II femoral neck fractures are treated with open reduction and internal stabilization using multiple lag screws placed in parallel. These patients are typically kept foot-flat weight-bearing for 2 weeks after surgery and then weight-bearing as tolerated after that. Hip precautions, including no crossing of the legs, using a pillow between the legs if lying on one side, not internally rotating the leg, sitting only on elevated chairs or toilet seats to avoid flexing the hips to 90 degrees, and using assistive devices for activities of daily living (such as putting on socks) are all kept in place for 1 month.

Treatment of type III and IV femoral neck fractures remains a subject of some debate. Generally, reduction via either open or closed method with internal fixation in younger, active patients is the method of choice. In older, less active patients, primary THR is advocated. In addition, in patients with concomitant acetabular pathology, THR is considered (see subsection on THR in hip OA section).

Treatment of both stable and unstable intertrochanteric fractures is generally with open reduction and internal fixation using the sliding hip screw implant. During this procedure, secure placement of the hip screw within the proximal fragment within 1 cm of the subchondral bone is essential. Early mobilization after surgery is also important. Weight-bearing status is usually limited for 2 to 6 weeks after surgery. The fracture generally heals within the next 6 to 12 weeks.

■ Complications

The most serious complication from a hip fracture is thromboembolic disease leading to death. The risk of mortality is greatest within the first 4 to 6 months after the fracture. Lower extremity DVT and fatal PE range from 40% to 83% in patients who are not anticoagulated and from 4% to 38% in patients who are anticoagulated. For this reason, it is vital to promptly antico-agulate a patient with a hip fracture (see subsection on THR in hip OA section for a more complete discussion of anticoagulation). High-risk patients may require placement of an inferior vena cava filter.

Other potential complications include AVN (less common in intertrochanteric fractures), infection, degenerative joint disease, and recurrent dislocation.

High-Yield Surgical and Functional Anatomy

The knee is a hinge type of synovial joint with three articular surfaces. The femoral and tibial condyles articulate on the lateral and medial sides, and the patella and femur articulate in between. The quadriceps are the primary extensors of the knee and are innervated by the femoral nerve (L2,3,4). The hamstrings are the primary flexors of the knee and are innervated by branches of the sciatic nerve (L5,S1). The anterior and posterior cruciate ligaments are critical in preventing anterior and posterior displacement of the tibia on the femur. The medial and lateral collateral ligaments are vital for lateral stability of the knee. Although arthroscopic procedures are increasingly the standard of care for many knee operations, there are several open surgical approaches to the knee. The medial parapatellar approach is one of the more common open surgical approaches.

■ Medial Parapatellar Approach

The medial parapatellar surgical approach to the knee provides excellent exposure of most structures and is used for total knee replacement (TKR), medial meniscectomy, removal of loose bodies, ligamentous reconstruction, as well as other pathologies. The patella is easily palpated superficially. The patellar ligament attaches the inferior border of the patella to the tibial tubercle.

The tibial nerve characteristically branches from the sciatic nerve before the popliteal fossa. The tibial nerve then runs deep to the popliteal fascia, covered by the semimembranous muscle. The tibial nerve then traverses superficial to the popliteal vessels and runs deep to the gastrocnemius muscle. Injury to the tibial nerve results in an inability to plantarflex the foot.

The common peroneal nerve also characteristically branches from the sciatic nerve before the popliteal fossa. The common peroneal nerve follows the medial border of the biceps femoris muscle and then passes superficial to the lateral head of the gastrocnemius muscle before running over the posterior head of the fibula. Injury to the common peroneal nerve results in an inability to dorsiflex the foot or put the foot into eversion. This results in foot-drop. Patients with foot-drop will have a high-stepping gait in order to clear their feet so that their toes do not scrape the ground.

Osgood-Schlatter Disease

Osgood-Schlatter disease is a common cause of knee pain. It is typically seen in athletic boys around the ages of 12 to 14. There is a 21% incidence in athletic children as opposed to 4.5% in children with sedentary lifestyles. Recurrent microtrauma from repetitive stresses (such as from repeated running and/or jumping) occurs within the cartilage of the tibial tubercle. Forty percent of patients with Osgood-Schlatter disease have bilateral involvement.

■ Clinical Manifestations

The typical patient complains of a painful, sometimes swollen, bump on the anterior aspect of the tibial tubercle. The patient does not report a history of trauma precipitating the symptoms. Usually the patient will give a history of participation in a sport or other activity that involves running and jumping, and these activities exacerbate the symptoms.

Physical Examination

On physical examination, the anterior tibial tubercle is typically tender and swollen. Both active and passive range of motion may be restricted secondary to pain.

■ Diagnostic Evaluation

The diagnosis is primarily made by history and physical examination, but plain film radiographs, including anteroposterior (AP) and lateral views, are also usually obtained and reveal normal findings with evidence of soft tissue swelling anterior to the tibial tubercle.

■ Treatment

The primary modality of treatment is conservative, including activity modification, ice, nonsteroidal anti-inflammatory drugs (NSAIDs), and stretching and strengthening exercises for approximately 6 weeks. Importantly, activities are altered rather than eliminated so as to minimize pain and discomfort. A patellar tendon strap or protective brace for the tibial tubercle is an excellent adjunctive treatment. Steroid injections are generally not recommended for this disease. In most patients (more than 95%), symptoms may persist for 1 to 2 years and then mostly resolve as the patient achieves skeletal maturity. Ossicles have been found to develop in 32% of patients after skeletal maturity and, when symptomatic, may be excised.

Osteochondritis Dissecans

Osteochondritis dissecans (OCD) in the knee occurs 80% of the time on the posterolateral portion of the medial femoral condyle at the point where the patella makes contact in full extension, suggesting that repetitive trauma plays a role.

The average age of presentation of juvenile knee OCD is 11 to 13 years old. The average age of presentation of adult knee OCD is 17 to 36 years old. Males are affected twice as often as females.

■ Clinical Manifestations

The typical adult patient is an active 20-year-old male who presents with a vague and poorly defined history of aching or swelling in the knee. As the disease progresses, the patient may complain that the knee "gives way." The patient may also complain of locking and/or catching. The symptoms are exacerbated with activity.

Physical Examination

Two features on physical examination are characteristic of knee OCD. The first is tenderness that localizes to the posterolateral portion of the medial femoral condyle. The second is a positive Wilson's sign, which is elicited by instructing the patient to lie supine with the knee flexed to 90 degrees. The knee is then passively internally rotated and slowly extended. As the knee is extended to approximately 30 degrees of flexion, the tibial spine abuts the OCD lesion on the medial femoral condyle, producing pain. This is a positive Wilson's sign. External rotation moves the tibial spine away from the OCD lesion and therefore should relieve the pain.

■ Diagnostic Evaluation

Plain film radiographs, including AP, lateral, and a notch or tunnel view, are obtained. Magnetic resonance imaging (MRI) is useful in order to delineate the size of the lesion, amount of subchondral involvement in the lesion, and quality of the articular surface. Asymptomatic lesions may occur, and therefore it is always important to correlate symptoms with radiographic findings.

■ Treatment

When selecting a treatment approach, it is important to consider the age of the patient, skeletal maturity, and qualities of the lesion. In skeletally immature patients with symptomatic lesions, conservative management should be employed for about 3 months. Conservative care for OCD in the knee includes limitation of activity with a knee immobilizer and protected weight-bearing. Full activity may be resumed once symptoms have abated and there is radiographic evidence of healing.

Skeletally immature patients who fail conservative care and adult patients with symptomatic lesions should be offered a surgical intervention. Surgical options include arthroscopic subchondral drilling, arthroscopic debridement and fragment stabilization, arthroscopic removal of loose bodies, open removal of loose bodies, and autologous chondrocyte transplantation (which is used primarily for extensive defects that have failed previous treatment).

Anterior Cruciate Ligament Injury

The anterior cruciate ligament (ACL) is commonly injured during twisting movements that classically result in an audible "pop." The typical patient is active and reports a history of participating in a sport or activity in which the patient rapidly decelerated or twisted a knee. Between 30% and 50% of patients will report actually hearing the "pop" at the time of injury. The patient may complain of subsequent buckling of the knee. Immediately following the injury, swelling of the knee is noted. If the patient has suffered a complete tear, the patient may report only minimal pain and often the ability to continue to walk or run. By contrast, patients with partial tears will typically complain of exquisite pain and significant morbidity.

Physical Examination
On physical examination, swelling is more pronounced in partial tears. This occurs because hemorrhage from the injury is confined to the joint. In complete tears, the swelling is less obvious because the ruptured joint capsule allows diffusion of the hemorrhage.

The most sensitive test for an ACL tear is the Lachman test. In this test, the knee is flexed to 20 to 30 degrees and AP glide is evaluated by the examiner (Figure 7-1). The anterior draw test is another good test for evaluating a suspected ACL tear. In this test, the knee is flexed to 90 degrees with the feet placed flat on the table. The patient's feet are stabilized on the table by the examiner (the examiner will typically sit on the patient's feet) and AP glide is then evaluated. A few degrees of AP glide with a firm endpoint may be normal. However, a loose endpoint or excessive glide is considered positive for an ACL injury. The affected side should always be compared with the normal limb.

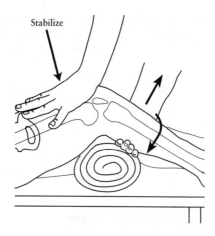

Figure 7-1 • The position of the examiner and patient for the Lachman test. It is very important that the patient be relaxed for this test. (Reproduced with permission from Gross, J. *Musculoskeletal Examination*, second edition. Figure 12.69, p. 369. Blackwell Publishing, 2002).

■ Diagnostic Evaluation

Plain film radiographs, including AP, lateral, and tunnel views, are used to evaluate an ACL tear in order to rule out a fracture. If a Segond fracture is found, in which the lateral tibial plateau is avulsed, this is pathognomic for an ACL injury.

Although not always necessary, MRI is a good imaging modality to assess for associated soft tissue pathology and to evaluate the extent of ACL injury.

■ Treatment

Primary treatment of an ACL injury includes controlling pain, encouraging early return to weight-bearing activities, and performing structured active range-of-motion exercises. The prognosis of an ACL injury depends on the frequency of buckling episodes, associated injury to the menisci and other ligaments, and the activities engaged in by the patient. For patients with small tears unassociated with other injuries, conservative care may be sufficient to restore adequate function. Bracing to improve function (including decreasing buckling episodes) may be offered to patients with more involved tears who wish to avoid surgery.

Surgical intervention is recommended for patients with an associated meniscal or ligament injury and for those who wish to return to participation in activities or sports with pivot movements (e.g., basketball) or side-to-side movements (e.g., skiing). Surgery is also offered to adolescents for whom activity restriction instructions are unlikely to be followed. There are benefits to earlier surgical intervention. Patients undergoing earlier surgery have been found to have fewer incidences of knee buckling and fewer incidences of progression to meniscal and articular injuries. Surgical options for ACL reconstruction include intra-articular (more common), extra-articular, and combined procedures. Early return to active and passive range-of-motion and weight-bearing exercises should be encouraged soon after ACL reconstruction.

■ Complications

Approximately 5% to 21% of ACL repairs require another operation as a result of the development of meniscal injuries, loss of motion, and/or hardware problems. Another potential complication from ACL reconstruction is arthrofibrosis, which may result when the reconstruction is performed too soon after the injury during the inflammatory phase.

Medial Collateral Ligament Injury

The medial collateral ligament (MCL) is typically injured by a valgus stress applied from the lateral side. This usually occurs during contact sports such as football, rugby, or soccer.

■ Clinical Manifestations

The typical patient is an active individual who reports a twisting injury with immediate subsequent swelling. The patient will often report having been tackled from the side during a contact sport.

Physical Examination

In the physical examination of the MCL, the knee must be examined in 30 degrees of flexion and then again in full extension. During provocative testing, the ankle is secured with one hand by the examiner and the other hand is placed around the patient's knee in such a way that the thenar eminence is against the fibular head and the fingers are able to palpate the joint line. The examiner then applies a valgus stress on the knee by moving the knee medially and the ankle laterally. By palpating the medial joint line during this maneuver, the examiner is able to assess the extent of gapping (Figure 7-2). Based on this evaluation, the degree of MCL injury may be graded. A grade I injury has 0 to 5 mm of medial opening. A grade II injury has 6 to 10 mm of medial opening. A grade III injury has 11 to 15 mm of medial opening.

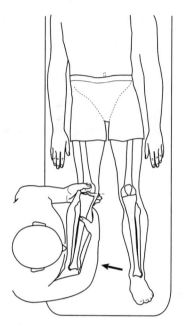

Figure 7-2 • Valgus strain (medial gapping). (Reproduced with permission from Gross, J. *Musculoskeletal Examination,* second edition. Figure 12.45, p. 359. Blackwell Publishing, 2002).

An isolated MCL injury will manifest in excess joint gapping during testing at 30 degrees of flexion but *not* in full extension. Excess joint gapping during provocative testing in full extension indicates that one or more cruciate ligaments may also be injured. The affected limb should always be compared with the unaffected limb.

■ Diagnostic Evaluation

Plain film radiographs are generally not indicated in suspected MCL injury. MRI is an accurate imaging modality to identify MCL injuries, but in the presence of a good physical examination, MRI is often unnecessary.

■ Treatment

Surgical intervention is not generally recommended for MCL injuries. Treatment is typically with a hinged knee brace. Physical therapy with early range-of-motion exercises and stretching and strengthening exercises are important components for healing.

Patients may be instructed that in an isolated grade I injury, the average return to full activities is approximately 2 weeks. For patients with an isolated grade II injury, the average return to full activities is approximately 3 weeks. For an isolated grade III injury, the average return to full activities is between 6 and 8 weeks.

Posterior Cruciate Ligament Injury

The posterior cruciate ligament (PCL) is often injured via a mechanism similar to a patella fracture, by an anterior stress placed on the lower limb. In PCL injuries, this stress is in the form of a blow to the anterior tibia, as in a motor vehicle accident in which the tibia hits the dashboard (dashboard injury). In athletics, a hyperflexion injury may also cause a PCL injury.

■ Clinical Manifestations

The typical patient will report being involved in either a motor vehicle accident or a hyperflexion injury with the foot in plantarflexion at the time of injury (e.g., sliding into a base and jamming the knee into the base).

Physical Examination

During the physical examination, inspection should evaluate the relationship of the tibia to the medial femoral condyle. The normal relationship between these two structures is that the tibial plateau is anterior to the medial femoral condyle. With a PCL injury, the tibia may subluxate and lie posterior to or be aligned with the medial femoral condyle.

A good clinical test tool for identifying PCL injuries is the posterior drawer test. The patient's feet are stabilized as in the anterior drawer test, but in the posterior draw test AP glide is tested by placing a posteriorly directed force on the tibia. If the tibia is able to glide abnormally backward on the femur, or if there is no firm endpoint to the glide, then PCL injury should be strongly considered. As always, the test should be repeated on the unaffected limb and the results of the two sides should be compared.

■ Diagnostic Evaluation

Plain film radiographs, including AP, AP weight-bearing, lateral, and tunnel views, should be obtained. The film is often normal but may reveal a bony avulsion fragment. This is important information because it will affect the treatment approach. MRI is highly sensitive and specific for PCL injury but is not routinely indicated if the physical examination is diagnostic.

■ Treatment

Most PCL injuries may be managed nonsurgically, with physical therapy used to emphasize quadriceps strengthening and stretching exercises. More severe PCL injuries may require surgical intervention using arthroscopic transtibial reconstruction, double bundle reconstruction, or tibial inlay reconstruction. PCL injuries that are associated with bony avulsion fragments require surgical treatment.

The postoperative rehabilitation plan is followed more cautiously than that for ACL reconstruction. Exercises to be avoided after PCL repair include knee extension against gravity and hamstring exercises. Bracing in full extension and quadriceps stretching and strengthening exercises should be pursued as the rehabilitation process progresses.

Meniscus Injuries

The roles of the menisci include contributing to the stability of the knee, facilitating and controlling the movements of the knee joint, and absorbing and distributing the body's load during movement. Ninety percent of the load during weight-bearing is carried by the medial compartment. This load-bearing burden of the medial compartment, combined with the fact that the medial meniscus is attached to the capsule and therefore less mobile, helps explain why the medial meniscus is torn three times as often as the lateral meniscus. The lateral meniscus has significantly less weight-bearing responsibilities and is not attached to the capsule, making it more mobile.

Seventy-five percent of meniscal tears are vertically oriented. A "bucket-handle" lesion occurs when a vertical fragment remains attached in the front and back. An anterior horn tear occurs if the tear emerges at the free edge of the meniscus and leaves an anterior tongue. A posterior horn tear leaves a posterior tongue. Horizontal tears are less common and are associated with degenerative tears in older patients.

The outer third of the meniscus receives its vascular supply from the capsule and thus has the potential for spontaneous recovery. However, because the remaining meniscus does not have a vascular supply, spontaneous healing of the tears in these regions does not occur.

■ Clinical Manifestations

The typical younger patient is an active individual who twists the knee during a sporting event. Pain (most often medial) is often intense and limits further activity. Swelling, when it occurs, generally does *not* occur immediately after the injury (as in ligament injuries) but several hours later. Sometimes the patient will complain of the knee locking in partial flexion or giving way spontaneously. Resting alleviates the symptoms, but when the patient returns to activities, even trivial twisting in the knee joint may precipitate similar symptoms. Sometimes the symptoms recur without any precipitating event.

The typical older patient may not report any precipitating injury before the onset of symptoms. Instead, the history may only be remarkable for the insidious onset of knee pain, giving way, and/or locking.

Physical Examination

On physical examination, an effusion may be present. The medial joint line will be tender in a medial meniscus injury, and the lateral joint line will be tender in a lateral meniscus injury. When the patient is instructed to flex and extend the knee, an audible or palpable click may be appreciated.

APLEY TEST

The Apley compression and distraction test is an excellent test for a meniscal injury. In this test, the patient lies in the prone position. The examiner flexes one leg to 90 degrees and, while stabilizing the back of the patient's thigh, the examiner leans on the heel of the patient's flexed leg to compress the medial and lateral menisci between the tibia and femur. The leg is then rotated into internal and external rotation while the compression force is maintained (Figure 7-3 A). When pain on the medial side of the knee is elicited with this maneuver, a medial meniscal tear is implicated. When pain on the lateral side of the knee is elicited, a lateral tear is implicated. While in the same position, the examiner then stops compressing the menisci and instead applies traction force to the leg while again putting the leg into internal and external rotation (Figure 7-3 B). The traction force reduces the pressure on the menisci and puts the pressure on the ligaments. If only the menisci are damaged, there should be no pain during traction (distraction test). If the ligaments are damaged in addition to the menisci, there may be pain with the distraction test.

MCMURRAY TEST

The McMurray test is helpful to identify a tear in the posterior half of the medial meniscus. In this test, the patient lies in the supine position with both legs in the neutral position. The examiner moves the patient's leg into maximal flexion. While palpating the joint line with one hand, the examiner rotates the patient's leg (using the ankle as a fulcrum) to loosen the knee joint. The examiner than applies a valgus stress and externally rotates the leg. Maintaining the valgus stress and external rotation, the examiner

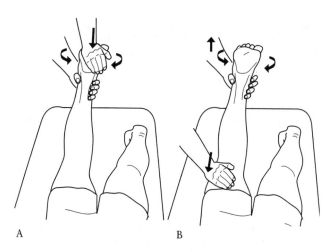

A   B

Figure 7-3 • The grinding/distraction test of Apley. The tibia is compressed first (A), then rotated while compression force is maintained (B). Distraction with rotation tests the collateral ligaments, whereas compression with rotation tests the menisci. (Reproduced with permission from Gross, J. *Musculoskeletal Examination*, second edition. Figure 12.76, p. 375. Blackwell Publishing, 2002).

slowly extends the leg while palpating the medial joint line (Figure 7-4). A positive McMurray's test is encountered when a palpable or audible click within the joint line is elicited during this maneuver.

■ Diagnostic Evaluation

MRI is the imaging modality of choice for investigating a suspected meniscal injury.

■ Treatment

Tears that are 10 mm or smaller, partial-thickness tears, and radial tears that are 3 mm or smaller are considered stable and do not require surgery. These tears merit initial conservative management consisting of NSAIDs, ice, activity modification, and a structured physical therapy program including strengthening and stretching exercises.

For more significant tears and tears that fail a trial of conservative treatment, surgical intervention is indicated. Surgical options include arthroscopic meniscectomy and meniscus repair. Partial meniscectomy is recommended for tears in the avascular region of the meniscus. Arthroscopic meniscus repairs with fixation are recommended for tears in the vascular region using the outside-in, inside-out, or all-inside method.

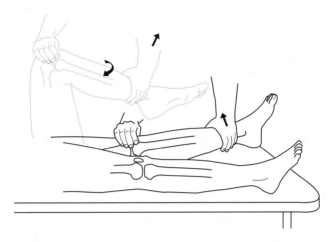

Figure 7-4 • McMurray's test is performed with the leg externally rotated and applying a valgus stress to test the medial meniscus. (Reproduced with permission from Gross, J. *Musculoskeletal Examination,* second edition. Figure 12.74A, p. 359. Blackwell Publishing, 2002).

Following a partial menisectomy, postsurgical rehabilitation includes physical therapy consisting of low-impact or nonimpact exercises, such as stationary cycling or straight-leg raising, beginning on the first day postop. Activities may be rapidly advanced to include all presurgical activities.

Physical therapy following a meniscus repair is longer and more intensive. Avoidance of weight-bearing with full range-of-motion exercises for 4 to 6 weeks postop is standard. Patients may be instructed that running is typically restricted until 4 months postop with return to sports after 9 months.

Knee Osteoarthritis

Knee osteoarthritis (OA) is a major source of morbidity. As with OA in other parts of the body, knee OA most commonly affects the elderly. For a more comprehensive discussion of OA, please see the section on hip OA. Osteoarthritic destruction of the knee appears in the radiographs of approximately 40% of 40-year-old patients. Knee OA is the most common underlying indication for a TKR.

■ Clinical Manifestations

The typical patient is older than age 40 and complains of knee pain that is worse with weight-bearing activity and better with rest.

The pain is often accompanied by stiffness and swelling. Morning stiffness typically lasts less than 30 minutes. Patients will also complain of the "gel phenomenon" in which stiffness occurs with inactivity and is relieved gradually with movement. In addition, the patient may complain of locking or giving way. Night pain is a serious sign and a significant indicator of progression of disease.

Physical Examination

Patients may have an obvious limp on physical exam. Localized tenderness in the knee may be present. Crepitus is typically also appreciated.

■ Diagnostic Evaluation

Plain radiographs should be obtained, including a standard AP view, lateral view, 45-degree posteroanterior (PA) view, and a skyline view of the patella. Typical signs include loss of joint space, subchondral sclerosis, cysts, and osteophytes (Figure 7-5). These findings must always be correlated with clinical exam because, as

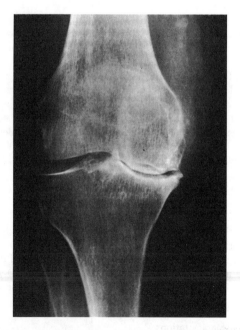

Figure 7-5 · X-ray appearance of osteoarthritis of the knee. (Reproduced with permission from Duckworth, T. *Lecture Notes on Orthopaedics and Fractures*, third edition. Figure 47.5, p. 375. Blackwell Publishing, 1995).

with other joints in the body, incidental asymptomatic osteo-arthritic findings on radiographs of the knee are common. If the diagnosis is uncertain, other diagnostic tools include computed tomography (CT), MRI, and arthrocentesis.

■ Treatment

Treatment of knee OA is based primarily on symptoms and comorbidities. Initial conservative measures include losing weight (when appropriate), strengthening and flexibility programs, non-impact exercises such as swimming, acetaminophen, NSAIDs, heat modalities, and rest. Topical analgesic therapy with methyl-salicylate or capsaicin cream may be beneficial. Glucosamine sulfate (1500 mg) and chondroitin sulfate (1200 mg) taken once a day has also been demonstrated to be helpful. Another conservative intervention is intra-articular injections of hyaluronic acid, which improve symptoms temporarily and usually need to be repeated periodically (about every 6 months).

In patients with persistent significant symptoms despite aggressive conservative care, surgery should be considered. Arthroscopy is less invasive than most surgeries and does not interfere with the potential for performing other future surgical procedures. Arthroscopy may be used to debride loose articular cartilage, implant cartilage in eburnated subchondral bone, and remove any loose bodies. After arthroscopy, patients may require the use of crutches for about 1 week while they are enrolled in a stretching and strengthening physical therapy program.

In younger, active patients who want to maintain an active lifestyle, osteotomy is another surgical alternative. The principle of osteotomy is to refocus the weight burden from the diseased medial aspect of the knee to the lateral side. Osteotomy is contraindicated in patients who cannot flex their knee to 90 degrees or who have more than 15 to 20 degrees of varus deformity. Following osteotomy, partial weight-bearing status is maintained until the bone has healed.

For patients with moderate or severe persistent symptoms from knee OA, TKR is an excellent alternative to improve quality of life.

Total Knee Replacement

In this procedure, the joint surface is removed and a metal and plastic prosthesis is inserted. Cement fixation, cementless fixation, and hybrid fixation designs are available. In TKR, cement fixation is the most common.

Following surgery, if cement fixation is used, then the patient is given weight-bearing as tolerated status. If cement fixation is not used, the patient is made toe-touch weight-bearing for approximately 6 weeks. After a TKR, strengthening exercises, range-of-motion exercises, and progressive ambulation are begun. Continuous passive motion (CPM) machines may also be used to facilitate recovery. Patients should target 90 degrees of knee flexion, which is required in order to enable activities of daily living such as sitting. Patients who have had a cement replacement may anticipate a gradual return to activity over the course of 1 to 3 months.

Complications from a TKR include deep vein thrombosis. Approximately 47% to 64% of patients who are not anticoagulated after surgery develop a clot. That number drops substantially to 6% to 24% in patients who are anticoagulated. (See the subsection on THR in the hip OA section for a more complete discussion of anticoagulation.)

Patellofemoral Disorders

Knee pain that is patellofemoral in origin is one of the most common presenting musculoskeletal complaints, and it represents a special challenge to physicians. Because a causative pathologic lesion is not always identified in patellofemoral disorders, it is particularly important to rule out referred pain from the hip for these patients (especially in adolescents who may have Legg-Calvé-Perthes disease or slipped capital femoral epiphysis). The causes of patellofemoral pain may be divided into four categories: (1) soft-tissue abnormalities, (2) patellar instability, (3) patellofemoral degeneration, and (4) idiopathic chondromalacia. Taken together, pain of patellofemoral origin may affect as many as 25% of all athletes.

■ Clinical Manifestations

The typical patient complains of knee pain that is classically dull and aching but may be sharp. The pain is usually in the anterior knee, but pain may be present in the retropatellar, peripatellar, or global knee. The patient will usually report that activities such as climbing or descending stairs, squatting, or prolonged sitting (movie theatre sign) exacerbate symptoms. Patients rarely report a history of trauma, but a trauma such as a motor vehicle accident in which the knee hits the dashboard could result in patellar subluxation or dislocation, which could precipitate patellofemoral pain.

Physical Examination
On physical examination, it is important to perform a complete examination of the knee and lower extremity, paying particular attention to the quadriceps angle (Q-angle). The Q-angle is formed

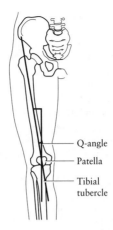

Figure 7-6 • Measurement of the Q-angle. (Reproduced with permission from Gross, J. *Musculoskeletal Examination,* second edition. Figure 12.12, p. 343. Blackwell Publishing, 2002).

by a line drawn from the anterior superior iliac spine to the midpatella, which is intersected by a line drawn from the midpatella to the tibial tubercle with the knee in full extension (Figure 7-6). The average Q-angle for females is 17 degrees, and the average for males is 14 degrees. The Q-angle is an indicator of patellar tracking. Patients with patellofemoral pain often have abnormal patellar tracking, reflected by an increased Q-angle on exam.

▓ Diagnostic Evaluation

Plain film radiography, with standard AP, lateral, and axilla views of the patella, is indicated. In adolescents a low threshold of suspicion should be used to order radiographs of the hip in order to help rule out underlying Legg-Calvé-Perthes disease or slipped capital femoral epiphysis. CT is sometimes ordered to assess for patellar alignment. MRI is not generally indicated except to rule out possible meniscal, articular, or ligamentous injury.

▓ Treatment

In most cases, patellofemoral disorders respond very well to a structured, supervised physical therapy program with an emphasis on stretching, strengthening, and proprioceptive exercises. Particular attention during physical therapy should be paid to strengthening the vastus medialis oblique in order to reduce lateral tracking of the patella. Patellar bracing and/or taping and

NSAIDs are also helpful. Activity is gradually advanced as tolerated. Once a patient is asymptomatic and has regained approximately 80% of preinjury strength, the patient may return to full activities. Returning to full activities with less than 80% strength will result in excessive guarding of the knee by the patient and will predispose to further injury. In patients who are not progressing well with physical therapy alone, an intra-articular corticosteroid injection may sometimes be helpful.

In the absence of an identifiable, correctable pathologic lesion, such as patellar tilt or instability, surgery should not generally be considered. Acute patellar dislocation is treated with closed reduction, aspiration of large hemarthrosis, temporary immobilization, and physical therapy. Acute disruption of the medial patellofemoral ligament is another indication for surgery in the form of an open repair. Isolated patellar tilt may be surgically corrected with an open or arthroscopic lateral release.

Patellar Fracture

Patella fractures are caused by direct or indirect trauma. An example of direct trauma is a motor vehicle accident in which the knee strikes the dashboard. Indirect trauma is characterized by eccentric muscle contraction during knee flexion. An example of indirect trauma is hiking in the wilderness, getting a foot stuck between two rocks, and then forcefully contracting the quadriceps in a futile attempt to free the foot.

■ Clinical Manifestations

The patient will give a history of either direct or indirect trauma with resulting pain and swelling over the patella.

Physical Examination

On physical examination, the knee will be swollen and tender. Occasionally there is an appreciable gap in the patella. If indirect trauma was the cause of the fracture, then straight-leg raising cannot be performed by the patient.

■ Diagnostic Evaluation

Plain radiographs, including AP, lateral, and Merchant views, should be obtained.

■ Treatment

For patellar fractures that are displaced less than 2 mm and have an intact extensor mechanism, conservative treatment is recommended, with early weight-bearing with the knee placed in full extension. A hinge brace is used for early active knee range-of-motion exercises.

In patellar fractures with more than 2 mm of fracture displacement and/or a dysfunctioning extensor mechanism (classically as a result of indirect trauma), open reduction with internal fixation is recommended. A partial or complete patellectomy is reserved for the rare case of a severe comminuted fracture.

Tibial Plateau Fracture

Tibial plateau fractures are classified using the Schatzker classification. Using this classification, types I, II, and III denote fractures involving exclusively the lateral tibial plateau. Type IV fractures involve the medial tibial plateau. Types V and VI are characterized by involvement of both the medial and lateral portions of the tibial plateau.

■ Clinical Manifestations

A pedestrian or bicyclist being struck by a car is a classic presenting patient history.

Physical Examination
On physical examination, there may be a large knee effusion, instability, bruising, and deformity. The surrounding soft tissues may feel like dough, which is caused by hemarthroses. It is important to perform a thorough neurologic and vascular examination of the entire lower limb to assess for associated injuries and to rule out compartment syndrome, which may present with severe pain, absent pulse, weakness, and/or skin pallor.

■ Diagnostic Evaluation

Plain film radiographs with AP, lateral, and AP with 10 degrees of caudal tilt should be obtained. A CT scan is useful to further delineate osseous defects. MRI may also be obtained in order to better assess the surrounding soft tissues.

■ Treatment

Minimally displaced tibial plateau fractures are treated with initial immobilization with a brace or cast. As the acute pain and swelling decrease, a hinge brace is instituted and structured range-of-motion exercises are performed. It is critical to maintain non-weight-bearing status until after radiographic evidence of bone healing has been observed. This typically takes between 8 and 12 weeks.

Severely displaced fractures, limb instability, open fractures, and compartment syndrome are all indications for prompt surgical intervention.

■ Complications

The peroneal nerve, popliteal artery, tibial nerve, and surrounding soft tissues may all be injured during the treatment of this injury.

8 Ankle and Foot

High-Yield Surgical and Functional Anatomy

The ankle is a hinge type of synovial joint. The ankle is composed of three bones: The talus bone articulates with the socket formed by the tibia (medially) and fibula (laterally). The fibrous capsule of the joint is strengthened laterally by the anterior talofibular ligament (ATFL, usually the first to be injured), the posterior talofibular ligament (PTFL), and the calcaneofibular ligament (CFL). The fibrous capsule is strengthened medially by the thick, strong medial deltoid ligament. The tibialis anterior muscle is innervated by the deep peroneal nerve (L4,5) and is the primary ankle dorsiflexor. The tibialis anterior also inverts the foot. The gastrocnemius and soleus muscles are the primary ankle plantar flexors and are innervated by the tibial nerve (S1,2). The numerous surgical approaches to the ankle include the anterior, medial, posteromedial, posterolateral, and lateral.

■ Anterior Approach

The anterior surgical approach to the ankle is used for draining ankle infections, removing loose bodies, treating fractures, and other pathologies. The superficial palpated structures include the medial malleolus, which is the distal medial end of the tibia. The lateral malleolus is the lateral distal end of the fibula.

The extensor hallucis longus extends the great toe. It arises from the anterior surface of the middle part of the fibula and attaches to the dorsal aspect of the distal phalanx of the great toe. It is innervated by the deep peroneal nerve. The integrity of the extensor hallucis longus is often used to evaluate the L5 nerve root.

The anterior tibial artery begins at the inferior border of the popliteus muscle and runs inferiorly between the extensor hallucis longus and tibialis anterior muscles, ending at the ankle joint, where it becomes the dorsalis pedis artery.

The medial malleolus surgical approach to the ankle can be reached via a more anterior or posterior approach. Typically, these approaches are used to treat fractures of the medial malleolus. The anterior approach offers excellent visualization of the medial malleolus but risks damaging the long saphenous vein and saphenous nerve running anterior to the malleolus. The posterior incision does not risk the saphenous vein or nerve.

Equinovarus Deformity

Equinovarus deformity (club foot) may be idiopathic, inherited through a polygenetic pattern of inheritance, associated with intrauterine malposition, or teratologic. Boys are affected twice as often as girls. In 33% of cases there is bilateral involvement.

■ Clinical Manifestations

The deformity of club foot is typically detected at birth. On exam the heel is found to be inverted, the forefoot adducted and supinated, and the ankle in equinus such that the sole of the foot is facing posteromedially.

■ Diagnostic Evaluation

The diagnosis is clinical, and radiographic evaluation is not usually necessary.

■ Treatment

Idiopathic cases of equinovarus may be treated with cast correction with or without Achilles tendon lengthening. Casting is continued from birth until 6 months. If, after 8 months, the patient still has the deformity, surgical intervention in the form of a full or partial posteromedial posterior ankle capsule release and release of the talonavicular, subtalar, and/or posterolateral tethers of the calcaneus is indicated. The degree of surgical release correlates directly with the degree and rigidity of deformity.

Teratologic cases of equinovarus are typically caused by spina bifida or other neuromuscular disease or syndromic osteochondrodysplasia. Radical posteromedial release is performed for patients with spina bifida. After release for these patients, it is critical that the talonavicular and subtalar joints be pinned in an adequate position. Prognosis is worse with higher spina bifida lesions.

Osteochondrodysplasias resulting in club foot are initially treated with casting. After casting, surgical release of the Achilles tendon, posterior tibialis and flexors, and capsular release may be required.

Ankle Sprain

Ankle sprains are the most common athletic injury. Figure 8-1 shows the different ankle ligaments. Almost all ankle sprains result from an inversion stress during ankle plantar flexion. Sixty to

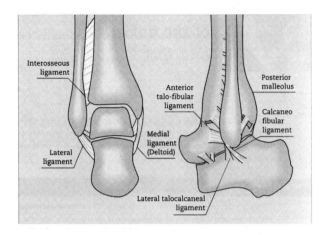

Figure 8-1 • Ligaments around the ankle joint. (Reproduced with permission from Duckworth, T. *Lecture Notes on Orthopaedics and Fractures,* third edition. Figure 20.1, p. 156. Blackwell Publishing, 1995).

■ TABLE 8-1	Grades of Ankle Sprain	
Grade	Description	Findings
I	Ligament stretched, but intact	No functional loss, able to bear weight and perform normal activities
II	Partial ligament tear	Difficulty with weight-bearing, able to perform most functional activities but with extreme pain
III	Complete rupture of the ligament	Unable to bear weight

seventy percent of all ankle sprains occur at the ATFL. Twenty percent of ankle sprains are combined ATFL and CFL or PTFL sprains. Table 8-1 lists the three grades of ankle sprain.

■ Clinical Manifestations

The typical patient is an athlete who reports having stumbled, inverting the foot beneath the body. See Table 8-1 for a description of typical findings associated with the different grades of ankle spain.

Physical Examination

On physical examination, a grade I sprain will be tender and have minor, if any, swelling. The anterior drawer test is performed by

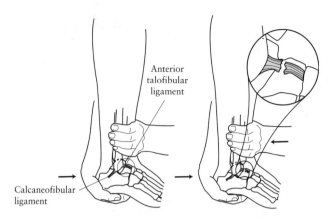

Figure 8-2 • Testing anterior drawer of the ankle. Excessive anterior movement of the foot indicates a tear of the anterior talofibular ligament. (Reproduced with permission from Gross, J. *Musculoskeletal Examination,* second edition. Figure 13.94, p. 424. Blackwell Publishing, 2002).

having the patient sit with both knees hanging over the edge of the examining table. The lower leg is stabilized by one hand of the examiner. With the other hand, the examiner takes the calcaneus and places the ankle in 20 degrees of plantar flexion before bringing the calcaneus and talus anteriorly (Figure 8-2). Excessive movement of the foot is a positive ankle anterior drawer test. A grade II sprain will reveal diffuse ligament tenderness and swelling. There may or may not be a positive anterior drawer sign. A grade III sprain will have significant pain, swelling, and a positive anterior drawer test.

■ Diagnostic Evaluation

The Ottawa ankle rules are a validated set of rules used for ankle injuries to eliminate unnecessary radiographs (Box 8-1). If the diagnosis is in doubt after radiographic evaluation, associated injury needs to be ruled out, or if surgery is considered, magnetic resonance imaging (MRI) may also be very helpful.

■ Treatment

Grade I and II ankle sprains are treated conservatively with bracing, rest, ice, elevation, early weight-bearing, and strengthening and range-of-motion exercises. Grade III sprains are typically treated initially with casting. Surgical intervention for grade III sprains remains controversial.

> ■ **BOX 8-1   Ottawa Ankle Rules**
>
> Using these rules, the following patients do not require radiographs:
> (1) Able to bear weight at the time of injury and able to ambulate four steps in the emergency room.
> (2) No tenderness over the medial and lateral malleoli.
> (3) No tenderness 6 cm superior to the medial and lateral malleoli.

Patients with ankle sprains often wish to return to their sport. Good conventional wisdom is that the patients may return to their sport when they are able to run, jump 10 times on the injured foot, stand on the injured foot for 1 minute with eyes closed, and pivot quickly on the injured foot without significant pain.

Most ankle sprains heal with conservative care, casting, or surgery. In patients with persistently symptomatic ankle sprains (failed ankle sprain), surgical repair of the ligaments may be required.

Achilles Tendon Injuries

The Achilles tendon may become inflamed (tendinitis), degenerate (tendinosis), subluxate, and/or rupture. Inflammation is typically caused by overuse in aging runners. Degeneration may be related to an underlying calcaneal bursitis. Subluxation or rupture is typically associated with a sudden stress to the tendon such as from a pushing-off movement.

■ Clinical Manifestations

The typical patient with Achilles tendinitis is a middle-aged male or female athlete, commonly a runner, who complains of gradually increasing pain in the Achilles tendon. The pain is exacerbated with repeated running and/or jumping.

The typical patient with an Achilles rupture is a middle-aged athlete who reports sudden pain and swelling in the Achilles tendon immediately following a pushing-off movement. The patient with an Achilles rupture may also report having experienced an audible "pop" or the sense of being "hit" across the posterior ankle with something at the time of injury.

On physical examination, the patient with Achilles tendinitis will have a tender Achilles tendon. The tenderness will shift as the tendon is passively and actively ranged through dorsiflexion and plantarflexion. Swelling and crepitus may also be noted. In patients with tendinosis, calcaneal tenderness is usually quite marked.

In patients with Achilles tendon subluxation or rupture, plantar flexion strength is limited and may be absent. The Thompson test may be used to evaluate for Achilles tendon rupture. In this test, the patient is placed in the prone position with the knee passively flexed. The calf of the patient is then squeezed by the examiner. This squeeze should cause the patient's foot to go into plantar flexion. Failure of the foot to plantarflex is a positive Thompson's test and indicative of Achilles tendon rupture.

■ Diagnostic Evaluation

In most cases of tendinitis or tendinosis, imaging is not necessary. For patients with refractory tendinitis or tendinosis who are contemplating having surgery, MRI should be obtained to identify regions of intratendinous degeneration. Patients with suspected rupture require lateral radiographs to rule out the possibility of posterosuperior calcaneal tuberosity avulsion. MRI should also be obtained in these patients.

■ Treatment

Achilles tendinitis is treated conservatively with rest, non-steroidal anti-inflammatory drugs (NSAIDs), orthotics (including insoles and support), and ice. Stretching and gradual strengthening with slow return to sport is also important for full recovery. In the few patients who do not respond to conservative care, longitudinal debridement of the tendon may be necessary.

Achilles tendinosis is treated with orthotics (e.g., heel lifts, heel pads), ionotophoresis, ice, and NSAIDs. Surgery is typically not indicated unless there is an associated Haglund's deformity, which is a benign cartilaginous growth at the posterior aspect of the calcaneus that may irritate the overlying bursa.

Achilles rupture may be treated with surgical or conservative management. A nonsurgical approach includes bracing. When bracing is pursued, ultrasound should be utilized to monitor progress. Surgery is often pursued in athletes wishing to return to their sport. Surgical approaches have been shown to increase range of motion and have quicker rates of return to sport than conservative approaches. Open procedures have been shown to have better outcomes when compared with percutaneous approaches. In addition, percutaneous approaches may be associated with sural nerve injury. Injury to the sural nerve during surgery may result in anesthesia or dysesthesia of the lateral foot.

Osteochondritis Dissecans

In the ankle, osteochondritis dissecans (OCD) occurs in the postero-medial aspect of the talus 56% of the time and in the anterolateral talus 44% of the time. In contrast to other parts of the body, OCD in the ankle is believed to be more frequently a result of trauma. However, controversy surrounds the pathophysiology of ankle OCD, with many authors believing that trauma plays a larger role in creating lateral ankle OCD than medial.

■ Clinical Manifestations

The typical patient is a male between the ages of 15 and 35. The patient may complain of ankle swelling, locking, and/or catching with walking. Approximately 90% of patients with lateral ankle OCD will report a history of trauma.

Physical Examination

The physical exam will reveal joint effusion, crepitus, and/or localized tenderness. Severity and the ability of the patient to localize symptoms to a specific point are associated with disease progression. It is also common for the patient to complain of pain when the examiner compresses the tibiotalar joint. Crepitus may be appreciated with active and passive dorsiflexion and plantar flexion.

■ Diagnostic Evaluation

Plain film radiographs, including weight-bearing anteroposterior (AP), lateral, and mortise views, should be obtained of the ankles bilaterally to exclude bilateral disease. MRI is also very useful in the evaluation, particularly in preoperative planning. Intra-articular injection of gadolinium increases the sensitivity and specificity of MRI for OCD.

■ Treatment

Patients with intact or only partially detached fragments may be treated with conservative management, including immobilization in a cast or brace and non-weight-bearing status for 6 to 12 weeks. Younger patients tend to respond better to conservative care. Patients with a medial lesion and a completely detached fragment still within the underlying crater bed may also merit conservative treatment for as long as 6 months. Patients with lateral lesions and a completely detached fragment require surgery. Surgical options are evolving and include arthroscopic subchondral drilling, arthroscopic debridement and fragment stabilization, removal of loose bodies, and autologous chondrocyte transplantation.

Anterior Bony Impingement

This disorder is common in dancers, basketball players, and football players. In fact, close to 60% of all dancers may experience this disorder. In this impingement syndrome, osteophytes occur on the anterior lip of the distal tibia and dorsal talar neck. Repetitive forced flexion places traction on the anterior joint capsule.

The osteophytes on the anterior tibial lip are classified based on the size and location of osteophyte. Type I are osteophytes smaller than 3 mm. Type II are osteophytes larger than 3 mm. Type III are significant bony exostosis with increased spur formation on the dorsal talar neck.

■ Clinical Manifestations

The typical patient is a dancer who complains of pain when landing from jumps or a football player complaining of increased dorsiflexion pain, catching, and swelling. On physical examination, swelling in the ankle joint is noted. Forced dorsiflexion may exacerbate the pain.

■ Diagnostic Evaluation

Plain film radiographs, including AP, lateral, and oblique views, should be obtained.

■ Treatment

Avoidance of excessive dorsiflexion, orthotics (e.g., heel lifts), NSAIDs, ice, and bracing may be used. In refractory cases, arthroscopic or open debridement may be necessary.

Plantar Fasciitis

Plantar fasciitis refers to inflammation of the thick band of fibrous tissue (the plantarfascia) on the plantar surface of the foot, and it is the most common cause of inferior heel pain.

■ Clinical Manifestations

The typical patient with plantar fasciitis will relate a history of insidious onset of medial plantar heel pain that often begins upon taking the first step of the day in the morning. Classically, the pain will alleviate after a few steps but tends to return later in the evening.

Physical Examination

On physical examination, point tenderness is elicited at the medial origin of the plantar fascia or along the distal portion of the plantar fascia. Passive dorsiflexion also elicits the patient's symptoms.

■ Diagnostic Evaluation

No imaging studies are necessary for this clinical diagnosis.

■ Treatment

The cornerstone of treatment is conservative care. Achilles tendon and plantar fascia stretching, activity modification, NSAIDs, orthotics (e.g., heel cushions and arch supports), night splints, and corticosteroid injections are all potential conservative measures. Activity modification, stretching, and orthotics are often all that is needed for successful treatment of this common disorder. If injecting corticosteroids, prudent care must be taken because atrophy of the plantar fat pad and rupture of the plantar fascia have been observed.

For the rare refractory case, cast immobilization for several weeks may be of benefit. Surgical intervention is rare and generally only indicated for persistent symptoms despite 6 to 9 months of aggressive conservative care.

Hallux Valgus

Hallux valgus is more common in women than men. Modern shoes with pointed toes are often to blame for this disorder in which there is pain at the medial eminence of the first metatarsal head (Figure 8-3).

■ Clinical Manifestations

The typical patient is a woman who wears pointed shoes and complains of pain at the medial eminence of the first metatarsal head that is worse when she is wearing her shoes, particularly after being on her feet all day.

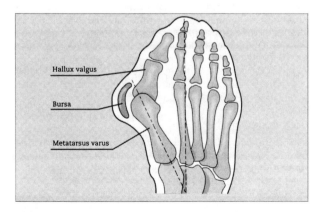

Figure 8-3 • Hallux valgus. (Reproduced with permission from Duckworth, T. *Lecture Notes on Orthopaedics and Fractures,* third edition. Figure 48.3, p. 386. Blackwell Publishing, 1995).

Physical Examination

On physical examination, there is an obvious tender prominence on the medial side of the first metatarsal head. There may be excessive mobility of the first metatarsocuneiform joint.

■ Diagnostic Evaluation

Weight-bearing plain film radiographs of the foot should be obtained. These films may show bony malalignment or arthrosis that will be otherwise missed with non-weight-bearing films.

■ Treatment

The primary treatment is usually conservative. Changing footwear to a wide, soft toe box and possible insertion of orthotics is often effective. Surgery is reserved for persistent pain or for diabetic patients with ulceration and foot neuropathy. There are many potential surgical procedures. Performing a distal first metatarsal osteotomy or a proximal first metatarsal osteotomy are among the most common. Complications with surgery include pain, stiffness, inadequate correction, and degenerative arthrosis.

Hallux Rigidus

This is a progressive degenerative disorder of the first metatarsophalangeal joint.

■ Clinical Manifestations

The typical patient will report a history of progressive pain at the top of the big toe. Occasionally the patient may recall a history of trauma precipitating the onset of symptoms. As the disease progresses and the patient shifts weight to take the load off the first digit, the patient may experience lateral foot pain.

Physical Examination

On physical examination, there is tenderness and pain with plantar and dorsiflexion. A tender dorsal osteophyte on the first metatarsophalangeal joint may be noted.

■ Diagnostic Evaluation

Plain film radiographs should be obtained and may reveal a flattened first metatarsal head, dorsal osteophytes, lateral squaring, and narrowing of the first metatarsophalangeal joint space.

■ Treatment

Conservative care emphasizes activity modification intended to decrease the load on the distal foot and redistribute it to the midfoot. Orthotics, including a rocker-bottom sole, may be of particular help. Dorsal cheilectomy is a preferred surgical option for treating refractory cases.

Interdigital Neuroma

This disorder affects women more commonly than men and is often a result of modern shoes with narrow toe boxes. The second and third interdigital spaces are most commonly affected. The interdigital nerve may be compressed and irritated beneath the intermetatarsal ligament. Wearing shoes with high heels or narrow toe boxes may compress the intermetatarsal ligament.

■ Clinical Manifestations

The typical patient is a woman who wears high-heeled shoes or shoes with narrow toe boxes and complains of numbness, tingling, or pain in the second or third web space. On physical examination, tenderness is localized to the involved interspace.

■ Diagnostic Evaluation

The diagnosis is usually clinical. Plain film radiographs may be obtained to rule out a stress fracture. When in doubt, a local anesthetic injection may be used for diagnosis. MRI or ultrasound may also be helpful.

■ Treatment

Conservative care includes changing shoes to a wide toe box, a metatarsal pad, a shoe with a rocker-bottom sole, and/or an interdigital corticosteroid injection. Surgical excision of the neuroma using either a plantar or dorsal approach may also be helpful. However, 20% of neuromas may recur after surgery. This failure rate may be the result of failure to completely excise the neuroma, recurrent neuroma, or the development of a stump neuroma from transecting the nerve.

Distal Tibial Fracture

Up to 25% of all physeal, or growth plate, fractures occur at the ankle. The distal tibial physis closes at about age 12 in girls and 13 in boys. The growing bone has four basic components (Figure 8-4). The diaphysis is the long part of the bone between the growing ends of the bone. The epiphysis is the most distal component of the bone in the direction of growth. Immediately proximal to the epiphysis is the physis. Proximal to the physis is the metaphysis, which is adjacent to the diaphysis. In growing children with open epiphysial plates, injury to the growth plate may result in growth

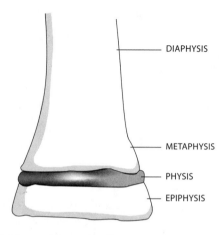

Figure 8-4 • Diagram of the anatomy of bone growth plate. (Reproduced with permission from Uzelac, A. *Blueprints Radiology,* second edition. Figure 8-5. Blackwell Publishing, 2006).

deficiencies. In children, the growth plates may be more likely to fail before failure occurs at the strong deltoid ligament or three lateral ligaments.

■ Clinical Manifestations

The typical patient is a boy or girl who is between 10 and 15 years old. The patient typically complains of pain and swelling at the site of injury. The patient often reports a history of injury while playing sports. On physical examination, swelling and tenderness is noted over the site of injury at the distal tibia.

■ Diagnostic Evaluation

Plain film radiographs, including AP, lateral, and oblique views, are obtained. Computed tomography (CT) is occasionally also obtained if the case is complex or intra-articular involvement is suspected but not proven by the plain films. Using the imaging studies, the fracture is classified based on the Salter-Harris classification (Figure 8-5 and Table 8-2). Type II is the most common, accounting for 75% of all cases (Figure 8-6 A and B); Type V is a rare fracture, accounting for less than 1% of all cases.

■ Treatment

The treatment of the fracture depends on the classification. A Salter-Harris type I distal tibia fracture that is nondisplaced is treated with initial immobilization in a short-leg walking cast for

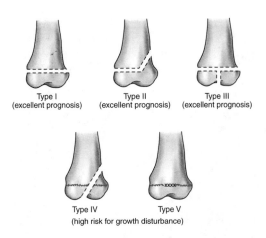

Type I
(excellent prognosis)

Type II
(excellent prognosis)

Type III
(excellent prognosis)

Type IV

Type V

(high risk for growth disturbance)

Figure 8-5 • Epiphyseal fractures: Salter-Harris classification. (Reproduced with permission from Uzelac, A. *Blueprints Radiology,* second edition. Figure 8-6. Blackwell Publishing, 2006).

TABLE 8-2	Salter-Harris Classification
Fracture Type	**Findings**
I	Displaced or "slipped" physis
II	Fracture above the physis, involving the metaphysis
III	Fracture below the physis, involving only the epiphysis
IV	Fracture through the metaphysis, physis, and epiphysis
V	Crush injuries to the physis

4 to 6 weeks. If the fracture is displaced, it is reduced and placed in a long-leg cast for 3 weeks with subsequent short-leg casting.

A Salter-Harris type II distal tibia fracture is treated with closed reduction followed by long-leg casting for 2 weeks with subsequent short-leg walking casting until union is achieved.

A Salter-Harris type III or IV distal tibia fracture is treated with closed reduction if the fracture is nondisplaced. If the fracture is displaced but can be reduced to within 2 mm, then it may be reduced via closed means as well. Percutaneous pin or cannulated screw fixation may also be used. Fractures that cannot be reduced via closed means require open reduction and internal fixation.

Salter-Harris type V distal tibia fractures are rare, and no formal recommendations are offered for treatment.

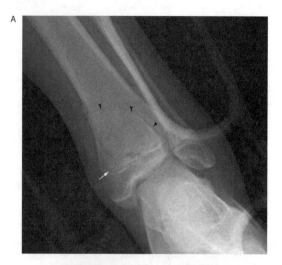

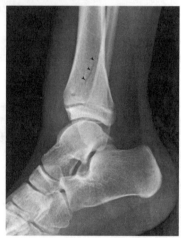

Figure 8-6 • (A) AP and (B) lateral views of Salter-Harris II fracture of the left ankle in a 12-year-old boy. The fracture line involves the distal tibial metaphysis. (Courtesy of Cedars-Sinai Medical Center, Los Angeles, California).

■ **Complications**

Salter Harris types I, II, and III distal tibial fractures in growing children all carry very good prognosis. Salter Harris types IV and V carry poor prognoses with a high risk for subsequent growth disturbances.

Calcaneal Fracture

The calcaneus is the most commonly fractured tarsal bone, accounting for 2% of all fractures. A calcaneus fracture usually follows a fall from a large height. On impact, the calcaneus is driven superiorly and is fractured against the talus.

■ Clinical Manifestations

The typical patient is a 45-year-old male who reports having fallen from a large height onto one or both of his heels. The heel is painful and swollen. Because the trauma precipitating the injury requires a large amount of energy, there are often concomitant injuries, and complaints of pain in the hip, spine, or pelvis are common.

Physical Examination

On physical examination, the heel is swollen, tender, and a contusion is noted. It is important to exam the hip, spine, and pelvis for associated injuries.

■ Diagnostic Evaluation

Plain film radiographs, including AP, lateral, oblique, axial, and Broden views, should be obtained. CT scans of the foot and ankle are also useful. In addition, a low threshold should be used to obtain radiographs of the hip, spine, and pelvis to rule out associated injury.

■ Treatment

If CT reveals less than 4 mm of displacement between the three facets, there is no subluxation, and no subfibular impingement is found, then the patient may be treated conservatively with temporary immobilization followed by compression hose and early range-of-motion exercises. Weight-bearing must be avoided for at least 12 weeks.

Patients requiring surgery generally require open reduction and internal fixation. This surgery is usually performed after swelling has decreased but before 3 weeks have passed from the time of injury.

Talus Fracture

The talus is rarely fractured. However, when a talus is fractured and not treated, the results may carry devastating long-term morbidity (Figure 8-7). The talus plays a pivotal role in linking the subtalar, transverse talar, and ankle joints. Sixty percent of the

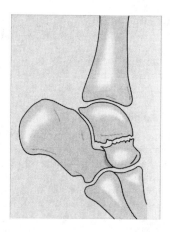

Figure 8-7 • Fracture of the talus reduced in plantar flexion of the foot. (Reproduced with permission from Duckworth, T. *Lecture Notes on Orthopaedics and Fractures,* third edition. Figure 20.9, p. 386. Blackwell Publishing, 1995).

talus is covered with articular cartilage. Fractures of the talus require large amounts of energy.

■ Clinical Manifestations

The typical patient will report a history of a significant fall precipitating the pain and swelling. On physical examination, there will be obvious deformity of the foot. It is important to check the neurovascular status of the foot in a patient with a suspected talus fracture.

■ Diagnostic Evaluation

Plain film radiographs, including AP, lateral, and oblique views, should be obtained. Hawkins classified the different types of talar fractures (Table 8-3). CT and/or MRI may also be helpful in the diagnostic evaluation, especially because there are often associated injuries.

■ Treatment

Treatment depends on the degree of injury. Hawkins type I fracture is treated with casting for 3 months and non-weight-bearing status for 1 month. Hawkins type II fracture is treated with closed reduction or open reduction and internal fixation. Hawkins type III is treated with open reduction and internal fixation. Type IV carries a poor prognosis and is treated with wound debridement.

TABLE 8-3	Hawkins Classification
Fracture Type	**Findings**
I	Nondisplaced fracture
II	Displaced fracture of the talar neck with subluxed or dislocated subtalar joint, and intact ankle alignment
III	Displaced talar neck fracture with dislocation of the talar body from both the subtalar joint and the ankle joint
IV	Includes a subtalar, tibiotalar, and talonavicular joint subluxation or dislocation

A salvage procedure may also be attempted for type IV injury. A talus-shaped methylmethacrylate spacer has been used with some success.

■ Complications

Avascular necrosis (AVN) is a serious potential complication of a talar fracture. Hawkins type I carries approximately a 10% risk of AVN, type II carries a 30% to 50% risk of AVN, and type III carries up to a 90% risk of AVN. Type IV fracture is associated with AVN and also an increased risk of infection.

A Opportunities in Orthopedics

Orthopedics is a surgical subspecialty that focuses on the surgical and nonsurgical management of diseases and injuries of the skeletal system and its joints, muscles, and associated structures. A residency in orthopedics involves 5 or 6 years (depending on the program and amount of research required) of postgraduate education. The first year of residency training is in general surgery. The remaining 4 or 5 years of training are in orthopedics and orthopedic subspecialties. After residency, many orthopedists pursue a fellowship in adult reconstruction, foot and ankle, hand, pediatrics, shoulder and elbow, spine, sports medicine, trauma, or oncology.

Orthopedics is an exciting, rewarding medical discipline. As such, it is a popular specialty with competitive residency slots. If you are contemplating pursuing an orthopedic residency, it is never too soon (or too late) to learn more. You can begin by talking to orthopedic residents and attendings. Ask them how they spend a typical day. Ask them what they like and don't like about their career decisions. Unfortunately, most medical schools do not allot elective time until either late in the third year or the beginning of the fourth year of medical school training. Try to rotate with an orthopedist during your general surgery rotation. Once you have elective time, do a rotation in orthopedics as soon as possible. But remember that a single good or bad orthopedic rotation does not necessarily translate into how you will enjoy your experience as a resident or attending in orthopedics. In the end, you need to put the whole picture together by talking to residents and attendings, doing rotations, reading, and exploring the advantages and disadvantages of orthopedics versus other medical specialties in which you might be interested. Orthopedics is a dynamic, interesting, stimulating field, but only you can decide if it is right for you.

Once you have decided that orthopedics is the specialty for you, it is time to consider your application. Residency directors are going to look closely at your grades and board scores, so study hard! However, another important factor is research experience. Participating in orthopedic research is a terrific way to learn about and contribute to the discipline. If you are considering orthopedics in your first or second year of medical school, that is not too early to get involved in a research project. If you don't come to orthopedics until your third or even fourth year of medical school, that's not too late to get involved with research. Talk to your advisors and discuss what aspect or aspects of orthopedics are most interesting to you. Next, find an orthopedist who conducts research that interests you and is interested in having your help. Then get involved and stay involved with his or her research project. Research is an excellent way to contribute to and learn about the field you will be entering. Involving yourself with a good research project will prove to be a rewarding experience. It will also give you a good topic of conversation during your residency interviews.

Finally, select one or two residency programs where you think you would be happy to work and where you think you would be a competitive candidate, and do orthopedic rotations at those institutions. During your rotation, learn as much as you can and ask questions. Doing a rotation enables the program to get to know you better and reciprocally enables you to get to know the program better. There are many excellent residency programs. Make sure that the residency program is a good fit for you. Some questions you will want to ask yourself include: Are the attending physicians invested in teaching? Are the residents learning? Are the residents happy with their program? Do the residents go on to fellowships from the program, and is that important to you? These are just some of the questions you should be asking yourself during your rotation.

QUESTIONS

1. A 46-year-old male patient complains of axial neck pain and right-sided scapular pain. The patient perceives the pain as deep and aching. The pain began 6 months after a motor vehicle accident in which the patient was the front passenger. The patient denies motor weakness, numbness, or burning. The patient has taken over-the-counter Advil for his pain with little relief. What is his likely diagnosis?

   A. Right cervical radiculopathy
   B. Atlanto-occipital dislocation
   C. Anterior cord syndrome
   D. Right cervical zygapophyseal joint disease
   E. Muscle strain

2. A 51-year-old female tennis player presents with 2 months of anterior shoulder pain that is more severe when she plays tennis. Her pain is relieved with rest. On exam, her shoulder is very tender, limiting both active and passive range of motion. On X-ray, a large calcification is seen just above the greater tuberosity. You diagnose her with calcific tendonitis and treat her for 6 weeks with a sling, modification of activities, NSAIDs, and heat. However, despite this treatment, her symptoms persist. The most appropriate next step in treatment is:

   A. Shoulder immobilization
   B. Intra-articular steroid injection
   C. Ultrasound-guided aspiration and lavage of the calcification
   D. Open surgical removal of the calcification
   E. Arthroscopic surgical removal of the calcification

3. A 46-year-old male plumber complains of right elbow pain that is worse at work. Recently, even picking up a pencil or the phone has become painful. The pain is located at the lateral epicondyle. On exam, resisted wrist extension reproduces the symptoms. What is the diagnosis and what is the first-line therapy?

   A. Ulnar collateral ligament injury: physical therapy, NSAIDs, rest
   B. Lateral epicondylitis: physical therapy, ultrasound, steroid injection, ice
   C. Ulnar collateral ligament injury: surgery

D. Lateral epicondylitis: surgery

E. Osteochondritis dissecans: arthroscopic lesion removal and abrasion chondroplasty

4. Kyphoplasty is used to treat:

A. Discogenic chronic low back pain

B. Lumbosacral radiculopathy

C. Osteoporotic vertebral compression fracture

D. Medial meniscus tear

E. Anterior cruciate ligament tear

5. A patient with a C5 radiculopathy will typically complain of:

A. Weak shoulder abduction, weak elbow flexion, numbness in her lateral arm and elbow

B. Weak shoulder abduction, weak elbow extension, numbness in her lateral arm and elbow

C. Weak elbow flexion, weak wrist extension, numbness in her fourth and fifth digits

D. Weak elbow flexion, weak elbow extension, numbness in her arm and third digit

E. Weak wrist flexion, weak finger flexion, numbness in her first three digits

6. A 62-year-old male presents with buttock pain that radiates down his lateral thigh into the top of his foot. He denies any weakness. He states that the pain is worse when leaning forward to tie his shoes. He denies any bowel or bladder changes, recent weight loss, or urinary symptoms. On exam there is no gait abnormality. Straight-leg raise reproduces his symptoms at 40 degrees of flexion. His extensor hallucis longus is weak compared to the unaffected side. His patellar and Achilles reflexes are brisk and symmetrical. This patient most likely has:

A. L4 radiculopathy

B. L5 radiculopathy

C. S1 radiculopathy

D. Zygapophyseal joint pain with a referral pain pattern in the leg

E. Discogenic low back pain

7. Cubital tunnel syndrome is a compression neuropathy of:

A. The median nerve at the elbow that results in numbness and tingling in the first three digits

B. The ulnar nerve at the elbow that results in numbness, tingling, and weakness in the first three digits

C. The ulnar nerve at the wrist that results in numbness and tingling in the fourth and fifth digits

D. The radial nerve at the elbow that results in numbness, tingling, and weakness in the fourth and fifth digits

E. The ulnar nerve at the elbow that results in numbness, tingling, and weakness in the fourth and fifth digits

8. In a patient diagnosed with slipped capital femoral epiphysis, the initial treatment consists of:

   A. Physical therapy, rest, and heat modalities
   B. Epidural steroid injection under fluoroscopic guidance
   C. Modification of activities, splinting, physical therapy
   D. Surgical intervention
   E. Physical therapy and/or intra-articular injection of hyaluronic acid

9. A 16-year-old female patient presents to the clinic complaining of right anterior knee pain. She denies any history of trauma. She is a dancer and the pain is worse with movement. On exam, the anterior tibial tubercle is tender. There is no joint line tenderness or restriction of movement. Her Q-angle is 16 degrees. She is able to squat on both feet, but this causes pain in her knee. The most likely diagnosis in this patient is: *Q angle is nml*

   A. Osteochondritis dissecans
   B. Anterior cruciate ligament injury
   C. Patellofemoral syndrome
   D. Osgood-Schlatter disease
   E. Osteoarthritis

10. A 40-year-old male presents with knee pain and swelling. He reports that the pain is mostly on the medial side of his knee. His symptoms began immediately after being tackled from the side during a weekend football game with friends. On exam, there is a normal Q-angle. There is excessive gapping when a valgus stress is applied to the knee in 30 degrees of flexion. There is no excessive gapping when the same valgus stress is applied with the knee in full extension. The most likely diagnosis in this patient is:

    A. Medial meniscal tear
    B. Anterior cruciate ligament tear
    C. Anterior cruciate ligament tear and medial collateral ligament tear
    D. Medial collateral ligament tear
    E. Posterior cruciate ligament tear

11. A type III Garden classification femoral neck fracture refers to:

    A. A valgus impaction of the femoral head
    B. A varus displacement of the femoral head
    C. A complete, nondisplaced fracture
    D. A complete loss of continuity between the fragments
    E. An avulsed fragment of bone

12. A 32-year-old male patient presents with a history of anterior shoulder pain that began 2 months ago. The pain is intermittent and is made worse by playing tennis. In the last week, the pain has kept him awake at night occasionally and prevents him from sleeping on his affected side. On exam, he has a positive Neer test and a negative

Speed test. The patient is able to abduct and slowly lower his arm without difficulty. The most likely diagnosis is:

A. Rotator cuff impingement
B. Rotator cuff partial-thickness tear
C. Rotator cuff full-thickness tear
D. Bicipital tendonitis *Speed test*
E. Acromioclavicular joint injury

13. In this test, the examiner flexes one leg to 90 degrees while stabilizing the back of the patient's thigh. The examiner leans on the heel of the patient to compress the medial and lateral menisci between the tibia and femur. The examiner then rotates the leg into internal and external rotation while maintaining a downward compression force. What is the name of this test, and what is it used to diagnose?

A. McMurray's test, meniscal tear
B. Wilson's test, meniscal tear
C. McMurray's test, collateral ligament tear
D. Wilson's test, collateral ligament tear
E. Apley compression test, meniscal tear

14. A grade III ankle sprain:

A. Involves only a stretch of the ligament
B. Is a complete rupture of the ligament
C. Is a partial ligament tear
D. Is a crush injury
E. Is a complete tear of at least two ligaments

15. A 43-year-old female presents with a complaint of wrist pain for the last 2 days. On further questioning, she reveals that the pain is on the radial side of her wrist and began shortly after gardening for the first time in years. On exam, there is tenderness over the tip of the radial styloid. She has a positive Finkelstein's test. She is diagnosed with de Quervain's tenosynovitis. The most appropriate imaging studies to order are:

A. X-ray only
B. X-ray and MRI
C. X-ray and CT
D. MRI only
E. No imaging studies are necessary

16. A Salter-Harris type II fracture is:

A. A displaced or "slipped" physis
B. A fracture through the metaphysis, physis, and epiphysis
C. A fracture above the physis, involving the metaphysis
D. A fracture below the physis, involving only the epiphysis
E. A crush injury

17. Select the primary hip extensor muscle and its nerve innervation.

A. Gluteus medius, superior gluteal nerve
B. Gluteus medius, inferior gluteal nerve

C. Gluteus maximus, superior gluteal nerve

D. Gluteus maximus, inferior gluteal nerve

E. Gluteus maximus, obturator nerve

18. The three most common causes of chronic low back pain, in descending order, are:

A. Discogenic, sacroiliac, zygapophyseal

B. Myofascial, sacroiliac, discogenic

C. Discogenic, zygapophyseal, contracted hip flexors

D. Buckled ligamentum flavum, discogenic, contracted hip extensors

E. Discogenic, zygapophyseal, sacroiliac

19. Kienbock's disease is:

A. Avascular necrosis and collapse of the lunate

B. Avascular necrosis and collapse of the scaphoid

C. Avascular necrosis and collapse of the triquetrium

D. A distal radius fracture resulting from a fall onto an extended hand

E. A distal radius fracture with ulna dislocation after a traumatic event

20. The rotator cuff muscles are:

A. Supraspinatus, infraspinatus, teres major, teres minor

B. Supraspinatus, infraspinatus, teres major, subscapularis

C. Supraspinatus, teres minor, subscapularis

D. Deltoid, supraspinatus, infraspinatus, teres minor

E. Supraspinatus, infraspinatus, teres minor, subscapularis

21. A 32-year-old female presents with complaint of wrist pain. She states the pain began after falling onto her outstretched hand 5 days ago. She was hoping the pain would go away on its own, but when it did not resolve she decided to come to the clinic. You palpate her wrist and find tenderness in the anatomic snuff box. You order plain film radiographs and a CT scan. Your diagnosis of a scaphoid fracture is confirmed. The fracture is displaced. Select the most appropriate initial management.

A. Open reduction and internal fixation

B. Closed reduction

C. A splint for 6 weeks followed by repeat radiograph and/or CT scan

D. No treatment. Close observation and follow-up are all that is needed.

E. Ice and physical therapy with early mobilization of the wrist joint to avoid contracture

22. Following a posterior approach for a hip replacement, hip precautions include:

A. No hip flexion past 90 degrees, no hip abduction beyond neutral, and no hip internal rotation past neutral

B. No hip flexion past 90 degrees, no hip adduction beyond neutral, and no hip internal rotation past neutral

C. No hip extension past 30 degrees, no hip abduction beyond neutral, and no hip internal rotation past neutral

D. No hip extension past 30 degrees, no hip abduction past 20 degrees, and no internal rotation past neutral

E. No hip flexion past 90 degrees, no hip adduction beyond neutral, and no hip external rotation

23. Accidental damage to the tibial nerve during dissection of the posterior knee may result in:

A. Weak knee extension
B. Weak knee flexion
C. Weak ankle dorsiflexion
D. Weak ankle plantar flexion
E. Weak extensor hallucis longus

24. A 26-year-old female presents with complaint of knee pain. The pain is described as dull and aching and located primarily in the anterior knee. She states that the pain is worse when she goes down stairs or sits for a prolonged period. She denies any history of knee trauma. On exam, her Q-angle is measured to be 20 degrees and the patella shows some abnormal lateral tracking. The joint line is not tender. There is retropatellar tenderness. Slight crepitus is appreciated with knee flexion and extension. Based on the information given, the most likely diagnosis is:

A. Osgood-Schlatter disease
B. Patella fracture
C. Medial meniscus injury
D. Early knee osteoarthritis
E. Patellofemoral syndrome

25. The platysma is a superficial muscle in the _____, and it is innervated by the _____.

A. neck, axillary nerve
B. neck, cranial nerve VII
C. shoulder, facial nerve
D. forearm, median nerve
E. forearm, radial nerve

26. A football player sustains an injury after falling onto his shoulder. Immediately following the injury, the player reports that his shoulder became painful and swollen over the end of the clavicle. On examination, focal tenderness is revealed over the clavicle, and the patient has difficulty adducting his arm across his body. If this patient has sustained a type I acromioclavicular injury, plain film radiography will reveal:

A. No displacement of the clavicle
B. Up to 25% displacement of the clavicle with no increase in coracoclavicular distance
C. Up to 50% displacement with no increase in coracoclavicular distance

D. Up to 50% displacement with an increase in coracoclavicular distance

E. Greater than 50% displacement with emergent surgery indicated

27. A 38-year-old woman presents with numbness and tingling in her first three digits. She also reports a vague aching sensation in her wrist. On further questioning, the patient reports that her symptoms are worse while typing at her desk. You suspect that this patient may have carpal tunnel syndrome. The most sensitive physical examination test for carpal tunnel syndrome is:

A. Tinel's sign
B. Phalen's test
C. McMurray's test
D. compression test
E. Finkelstein's test

28. Using provocative discogram with post-discogram CT evaluation to evaluate for discogenic back pain, a grade III fissure in the annulus fibrosus refers to a fissure that penetrates:

A. The inner third of the annulus
B. The inner half of the annulus
C. The outer third of the annulus
D. Circumferentially around less than half of the rim of the annulus
E. Circumferentially around the rim of the annulus

29. An infant is evaluated and found to have evidence of hip instability. The most appropriate diagnostic test is:

A. X-ray
B. CT
C. MRI with contrast
D. MRI without contrast
E. Ultrasonography

30. Injury to the common peroneal nerve results in decreased ability to:

A. Plantarflex the foot
B. To extend the knee and dorsiflex the foot
C. Flex the knee and dorsiflex the foot
D. Dorsiflex the foot and invert the foot
E. Dorsiflex the foot and evert the foot

31. A 36-year-old male presents with a complaint of slowly progressive right medial heel pain. The patient states that the pain is worst when he first wakes up and takes his first step of the day. On physical examination, there is no notable atrophy of the muscles. Reflexes are brisk and intact bilaterally. Passive dorsiflexion exacerbates the patient's symptoms. Based on the information provided, the first diagnostic imaging to order is:

A. X-ray
B. CT

    C. MRI
    D. Bone scan
    E. No imaging is necessary

32. The Hawkins test is used to evaluate for:

    A. Meniscus injury
    B. Posterior shoulder instability
    C. Biceps tendon instability
    D. Shoulder impingement syndrome
    E. Osteochondritis dissecans in the elbow

33. Supracondylar fractures are the most common type of pediatric elbow fracture. In the Gartland classification of supracondylar fractures, type II refers to:

    A. Anterior gapping with some rotational malalignment and an intact posterior hinge
    B. Anterior gapping with some rotational malalignment and an unstable posterior hinge
    C. Anterior gapping without rotational malalignment and an intact posterior hinge
    D. Anterior gapping without rotational malalignment and an unstable posterior hinge
    E. No anterior gapping and moderate rotational malalignment

34. The tendons of the extensor carpi radialis longus and extensor carpi radialis brevis muscles are found in the:

    A. First dorsal wrist tunnel
    B. Second dorsal wrist tunnel
    C. Third dorsal wrist tunnel
    D. Fourth dorsal wrist tunnel
    E. Fifth dorsal wrist tunnel

35. A young girl who is skeletally immature and has a scoliotic curve should be treated with full-time bracing if her curve is:

    A. Less than 10 degrees
    B. Between 10 and 20 degrees
    C. Between 20 and 40 degrees
    D. Greater than 60 degrees
    E. Full-time bracing is never appropriate in a skeletally immature adolescent

36. The quadriceps muscles include the:

    A. Rectus femoris, vastus lateralis, vastus medialis, iliopsoas
    B. Rectus femoris vastus lateralis, vastus medialis, biceps femoris
    C. Rectus femoris, biceps femoris, vastus intermedius, sartorius
    D. Biceps femoris, vastus lateralis, vastus medialis, vastus intermedius
    E. Rectus femoris, vastus lateralis, vastus medialis, vastus intermedius

37. A 14-year-old male presents with a complaint of a limp and left groin and knee pain. He states that the pain is dull and aching. He states he has no shooting pains, numbness, tingling, or burning. He cannot recall any history of trauma, but the pain does seem to be worse when he plays basketball. On physical examination, the patient is moderately overweight. Gait examination reveals out-toeing and a mildly antalgic gait pattern. When his hip is externally rotated, the patient tends to flex his hip. The most likely diagnosis is:

    A. Legg-Calvé-Perthes disease
    B. Axial low back pain with referral pain pattern
    C. L4 radiculopathy
    D. Transient synovitis
    E. Slipped capital femoral epiphysis

38. A 22-year-old male presents with a complaint of left knee pain. The pain is aching in quality. Occasionally, the patient reports that his knee catches and locks. The patient does not recall any history of his knee "giving out." The patient cannot recall any history of significant trauma except for a large bruise on his knee that he suffered after a football collision two years ago. On examination, the patient is instructed to lie on his back. His knee is flexed to 90 degrees and put into internal rotation and slowly extended. When his knee is at 30 degrees of flexion, he reports significant pain. With his knee still in 30 degrees of flexion, his knee is rotated into external rotation and the pain is relieved. This is called the _____ and it is diagnostic of _____.

    A. Wilson's sign, osteochondritis dissecans
    B. Wilson's sign, medial meniscus injury
    C. McMurray's test, lateral meniscus injury
    D. McMurray's test, osteochondritis dissecans
    E. Yergason's test, medial meniscus injury

39. Using the Schatzker classification, a tibial plateau fracture that involves only the medial tibial plateau is a:

    A. Type I fracture
    B. Type II fracture
    C. Type III fracture
    D. Type IV fracture
    E. Type V fracture

40. An infant is found to have an inverted left heel, forefoot adduction and supination, and the sole of the foot faces posteromedially. A clinical diagnosis of idiopathic club foot (equinovarus deformity) is made. The next appropriate step in the management of this patient is:

    A. Radiographic examination
    B. CT evaluation
    C. Casting with or without Achilles tendon lengthening
    D. No casting; proceed with immediate surgical correction
    E. MRI

41. A 33-year-old woman presents with a complaint of pain between the second and third web spaces of her right foot. On further questioning, she reports that the "pain" is really more of a burning sensation. There is tenderness over the involved web space. The most likely diagnosis is:

    A. Ganglion cyst
    B. Hallux valgus
    C. Stress fracture
    D. Interdigital neuroma
    E. L5 radicular pain

42. Monteggia fracture is characterized by:

    A. Isolated ulna fracture
    B. Proximal radius fracture and radial head dislocation
    C. Crush fracture of the distal ulna and radial head dislocation
    D. Distal ulna fracture and radial head dislocation
    E. Proximal ulna fracture and radial head dislocation

43. During a posterior approach to the hip, the sciatic nerve is most commonly found to be exiting:

    A. Below the piriformis
    B. Above the piriformis
    C. Through the gluteus maximus
    D. Through the obturator internus
    E. The sciatic nerve is not encountered in the posterior approach to the hip

44. The primary external rotator muscles of the shoulder are the infraspinatus and teres minor muscles. Respectively, these two muscles are innervated by the _____ nerve and the _____ nerve.

    A. suprascapular, subscapular
    B. subscapular, axillary
    C. suprascapular, axillary
    D. axillary, suprascapular
    E. suprascapular, subclavius

45. Injury to the median nerve during surgery of the elbow may result in loss of:

    A. Forearm pronation, wrist and digit extension, and thumb apposition
    B. Forearm supination, wrist and digit extension, and thumb apposition
    C. Forearm pronation, wrist extension, digit flexion, and thumb apposition
    D. Sensation on the lateral portion of the palm and the palmar part of the first three digits, loss of forearm pronation, and loss of wrist and digit extension
    E. Forearm pronation, wrist and digit flexion, and thumb apposition

46. A patient presents with shooting pain that radiates down the neck and arm into the hand. The examiner passively extends the patient's neck and rotates it to the painful side. The examiner then applies gentle axial compression to the top of the head. This is called the _____ and it is used to help diagnose _____.

    A. Johnson test, cervical radicular symptoms
    B. Johnson test, cervical zygapophyseal joint disease
    C. Spurling test, cervical radicular symptoms
    D. Spurling test, cervical zygapophyseal joint disease
    E. Spurling test, cervical spondylotic myelopathy

47. The O'Brien compression test is useful in differentiating a superior labral anterior posterior (SLAP) lesion and acromioclavicular (AC) joint disease. The O'Brien test is performed by having the patient stand with the shoulder flexed to 90 degrees and the elbow in full extension. Next, the shoulder is adducted 10 to 15 degrees and internally rotated so that the thumb points to the floor. From behind the patient, the examiner then applies a downward-directed force to the arm as the patient resists. The patient's hand is then supinated and the maneuver is repeated. The patient has a positive O'Brien test, suggesting a SLAP lesion, if:

    A. Pain is worse when the hand is in pronation, and provided that the pain is experienced in the AC joint
    B. Pain is worse when the hand is in pronation, and provided that the pain is experienced within the shoulder
    C. Pain is worse when the hand is in supination, and provided that the pain is experienced in the AC joint
    D. Pain is worse when the hand is in supination, and provided that the pain is experienced within the shoulder
    E. Pain is equally severe with the hand in supination and pronation, and the pain is experienced within the shoulder and radiates halfway down the lateral aspect of the arm

48. In contrast to other parts of the body, osteochondritis dissecans of the ankle is thought to be most likely caused by:

    A. Ischemia
    B. Trauma
    C. Genetics
    D. Idiopathic
    E. Radiation exposure

49. The Thompson test is used to evaluate for:

    A. Knee medial meniscus tear
    B. Hip flexor contraction
    C. Hip extensor contraction
    D. Achilles tendon rupture
    E. Achilles tendonitis

50. After a total hip replacement using polymethylmethacrylate cement for fixation, the patient may return to weight-bearing as tolerated:
    A. One day after surgery
    B. Two weeks after surgery
    C. Four weeks after surgery
    D. Six weeks after surgery if there is evidence of bone healing on radiographs
    E. No sooner than 8 weeks after surgery regardless of evidence of bone healing on radiographs

ANSWER KEY

1. D	14. B	27. D	40. C
2. C	15. E	28. C	41. D
3. B	16. C	29. E	42. E
4. C	17. D	30. E	43. A
5. A	18. E	31. E	44. C
6. B	19. A	32. D	45. E
7. E	20. E	33. A	46. C
8. D	21. A	34. B	47. D
9. D	22. B	35. C	48. B
10. D	23. D	36. E	49. D
11. B	24. E	37. E	50. A
12. A	25. B	38. A	
13. E	26. A	39. D	

ANSWERS

1. **D.** The case described is classic for cervical zygapophyseal joint disease causing axial neck pain with a referral pain pattern in the right scapula. Radiculopathy is characterized by a state of neurologic loss such as weakness or numbness. This patient does not complain of either. Radiculopathy is often accompanied by radicular pain, which is electric and radiates in a bandlike manner. This patient's pain is deep and aching, which is characteristic of referred pain. Patients with anterior cord syndrome typically complain of problems with balance and weakness in the lower extremities. Muscle strain is not a specific diagnosis, and straining a muscle would not account for this patient's 6-month duration of symptoms. Atlanto-occipital dislocation may occur after a motor vehicle accident, but patients are typically unresponsive.

2. **C.** This patient does have rotator cuff calcific tendonitis, and the most appropriate initial intervention was performed. At this point, the patient should undergo ultrasound-guided aspiration and lavage. This is a good, minimally invasive alternative to surgery. If this fails, surgical removal should be considered. Shoulder immobilization is inappropriate and could lead to further complications, such as adhesive capsulitis.

3. **B.** More than 95% of patients with lateral epicondylitis achieve satisfactory results from a combination of physical therapy, ultrasound, NSAIDs, rest, iontophoresis, electrical stimulation, and steroid injections.

4. **C.** Kyphoplasty is a procedure used for osteoporotic compression fracture where an inflatable bone tamp is inserted percutaneously into the vertebral body. The tamp is then inflated and used to help

inject polymethylmethacrylate under low pressure. Kyphoplasty is contraindicated if there is a defect in the posterior cortex of the vertebral body. Lumbosacral radiculopathy is generally treated initially with conservative measures such as physical therapy and epidural steroid injections. Surgery is indicated for progressive neurologic deficits and for persistent symptoms despite conservative care. Discogenic low back pain is treated with intradermal electrothermal annuloplasty, nucleoplasty, or fusion surgery. Medial meniscus tear and anterior cruciate ligament tear are injuries of the knee, which can be treated conservatively or surgically, depending on the extent of the injury.

5. **A.** C5 radiculopathy results in weak shoulder abduction (weak deltoid) and weak elbow flexion. Because elbow flexion receives greater input from C6, shoulder abduction is relatively weaker than elbow flexion. Burning, numbness, tingling, and shooting pain may radiate into the lateral arm and lateral elbow. Weak elbow extension and weak wrist flexion are characteristic of a C7 radiculopathy. Weak wrist extension is characteristic of a C6 radiculopathy. Weak finger flexion is characteristic of a C8 radiculopathy.

6. **B.** Radiating pain, numbness, and/or burning down the lateral thigh into the dorsum of the foot are classic for an L5 radiculolpathy. Patients will often also have a Trendelenburg gait caused by a weak gluteus medius. Patients also typically have a weak extensor hallucis longus (weak big toe extensor). Straight-leg raise is classically positive. Because this patient's pain is worse with forward flexion, he probably has a disc protrusion or herniation compressing the nerve root, causing inflammation and his symptoms. If extension worsened his symptoms, spinal stenosis would be more likely. In an L4 radiculopathy, patients complain of symptoms radiating down the anterior thigh, crossing the knee, into the anteromedial leg and medial malleolus. In addition, patients may complain of weakness with attempted leg extension. The patellar reflex may also be sluggish and asymmetric. In an S1 radiculopathy, patients complain of symptoms radiating down the posterior buttock, along the posterior thigh, and into the lateral malleolus and foot, including the web space between the fourth and fifth toes. The Achilles reflex may be sluggish and asymmetric. Plantar flexion may also be weak.

7. **E.** Cubital tunnel syndrome also results in a deep aching sensation in the elbow. The site of compression in the elbow is often between the two heads of the flexor carpi ulnaris. Small finger abduction and weakness is called Wartenberg's sign and is sometimes present. When the ulnar nerve is compressed in the tunnel of Guyon at the wrist, there is no numbness and tingling in the fourth and fifth digits because the ulnar nerve gives off the sensory branch to this area proximal to the wrist.

8. **D.** Slipped capital femoral epiphysis is one of the most common adolescent hip disorders and is a surgical emergency. Delay in treatment increases the risk of avascular necrosis.

9. **D.** This patient has a classic history for Osgood-Schlatter disease. The fact that her pain is worse with dancing and that she has tibial tubercle tenderness further supports the diagnosis. Patients with osteochondritis dissecans complain of their knee giving way and/or locking. Patients with anterior cruciate ligament injury describe a precipitating injury that is often associated with a "pop" and buckling of the knee. Patients with patellofemoral syndrome often have an abnormal Q-angle. The tibial tubercle would not be tender in a patient with patellofemoral syndrome. This patient is too young to have osteoarthritis unless there was a secondary cause. However, in this patient with a classic history and physical for Osgood-Schlatter disease, this diagnosis should be considered first.

10. **D.** Medial gapping during a valgus stress indicates a medial collateral ligament tear. When there is excessive gapping during valgus stress with the knee in 30 degrees of flexion but not in full extension, the tear is probably isolated to the medial collateral ligament. A meniscal tear does not typically present in this manner. Pain and swelling do not immediately precipitate the injury, and gapping would not be present.

11. **B.** Type I is valgus impaction of the femoral head. Type II is a complete, nondisplaced fracture. Type III is varus displacement of the femoral head. Type IV is complete loss of continuity between the fragments. Higher Garden classifications have a greater association with the subsequent development of avascular necrosis.

12. **A.** The patient has impingement of his rotator cuff. A positive Neer test is classic for impingement syndrome. The Speed test is used to assess for bicipital tendonitis. Because it is negative, and because bicipital tendon tenderness was not mentioned, it is less likely that the patient has bicipital tendonitis. Partial- or full-thickness tears of the rotator cuff would result in weakness. In a full-thickness tear, the drop-arm test would be positive. No history of trauma is given to make one suspicious of an acromioclavicular injury. A good way to further evaluate this patient would be to inject 10 mL of 1% lidocaine (or another anesthetic) into the subacromial space and to repeat the Neer test. After the injection, there should be no pain with the Neer test maneuver (in which the examiner stabilizes the scapula with one hand and flexes the patients shoulder with the other).

13. **E.** This describes the Apley compression test, which is used to help diagnose a meniscal tear. When it is positive, the Apley distraction test can be used to help differentiate a meniscal tear from a ligament tear. The Apley distraction test is performed in the same way as the compression test, except instead of the downward compression force, an upward distraction force is used. This maneuver unloads the pressure from the meniscus and should not be painful if only a meniscus is torn. If, however, a ligament is torn, then the maneuver will be painful. McMurray's test is also used to diagnose a meniscus injury. In McMurray's test, the examiner moves the

patient's leg into maximal flexion, applies a valgus stress, and externally rotates the leg. Maintaining the valgus stress and external rotation, the examiner slowly extends the leg while palpating the medial joint line. In a posterior medial meniscus injury, a palpable or audible click may be appreciated as the leg is extended in this position. Wilson's test is used to evaluate osteochondritis dissecans in the medial femoral condyle.

14. **B.** A grade I sprain is a stretch of the ligament but the ligament is still intact. A grade II sprain is a partial ligament tear. A grade III sprain is a complete rupture of the ligament. The most common ligament that is sprained in the ankle is the anterior talofibular ligament (ATFL). The second ligament to be sprained in the lateral ankle is the calcaneofibular ligament (CFL). A posterior talofibular (PTFL) sprain is rare and only occurs in severe sprains.

15. **E.** De Quervain's tenosynovitis is a clinical diagnosis. This patient's history and physical exam are classic for de Quervain's tenosynovitis. Finkelstein's test is positive when the patient's thumb is passively adducted across the palm, eliciting pain in the radial styloid. Patients may be treated with avoidance of the offending activity (gardening in this case), splinting, and/or steroid injection(s). Surgical unroofing of the first dorsal compartment is reserved for the infrequent recalcitrant case.

16. **C.** Salter-Harris type I is a displaced or "slipped" physis. Type II is the most common, accounting for 75% of all cases, and includes fractures above the physis, involving the metaphysis. Type III is a fracture below the physis, involving only the epiphysis. Type IV is a fracture through the metaphysis, physis, and epiphysis. Type V is a rare fracture, accounting for less than 1% of all cases, and includes crush injuries to the physis.

17. **D.** The primary hip extensor is the gluteus maximus, which is innervated by the inferior gluteal nerve (S1). The primary hip abductor is the gluteus medius, which is innervated by the superior gluteal nerve (L5). The obturator nerve innervates the adductor longus, which is the primary hip adductor.

18. **E.** Chronic low back pain is caused by a painful intervertebral disc (discogenic) in 39% of patients. It is caused by painful zygapophyseal joint disease in 15% of younger patients and as much as 40% of elderly patients. It is caused by sacroiliac joint disease in 15% of patients. Contracted hip flexors or extensors are not a proven source of chronic low back pain. Nevertheless, in chronic low back pain, flexor and extensor muscles may become contracted and should be evaluated and treated. However, an underlying source of the pain should also be sought.

19. **A.** Kienbock's disease is avascular necrosis and collapse of the lunate leading to carpal collapse. Ultimately, this disease progresses to generalized wrist arthrosis. Patients are typically young adults complaining of aching and stiffness in the wrist.

20. **E.** The rotator cuff muscles provide stability to the shoulder. The supraspinatus abducts the shoulder. The infraspinatus and teres minor externally rotate the shoulder. The subscapularis internally rotates the shoulder. The deltoid and teres major are not rotator cuff muscles.

21. **A.** A displaced scaphoid fracture must be treated urgently with open reduction and internal fixation to avoid avascular necrosis. A nondisplaced scaphoid fracture may be treated with strict immobilization. A scaphoid tubercle fracture may be treated as a wrist sprain with a bandage and early movement.

22. **B.** Patients are often instructed not to cross their legs, to use a pillow between their legs if lying on one side, and to not bend over to tie their shoes. Also, elevated toilet seats are useful. All of these instructions are to help the patient remember to not flex their hip past 90 degrees, not adduct their hip beyond neutral, and not internally rotate their hip past neutral. These hip precautions are followed for at least 1 month and are used to help avoid stressing the hip joint at the vulnerable posterior part of the capsule.

23. **D.** The tibial nerve branches from the sciatic nerve and innervates the gastrocnemius muscle and the soleus muscle. These are the two primary plantar flexors. Damage to the tibial nerve may therefore result in foot drop.

24. **E.** This patient's presentation is typical of patellofemoral syndrome. In Osgood-Schlatter disease, the patient would be younger and the history and/or exam would include tenderness in the tibial tuberosity. A patella fracture would follow a trauma such as a motor vehicle accident. A medial meniscus injury in a young patient is typically associated with a traumatic injury and joint line tenderness, and McMurray's or Apley compression tests would be positive. Early knee osteoarthritis is possible but rare and unlikely in this patient with no risk factors given. Because of the classic presentation and high prevalence, patellofemoral syndrome is the most likely diagnosis in this patient.

25. **B.** The platysma is a thin superficial muscle in the neck that tenses the skin and draws the corner of the mouth in an inferior direction. The platysma muscle is very important for facial expression. It is innervated by the seventh cranial nerve (also called the facial nerve).

26. **A.** A type I AC joint injury is characterized by a sprain of the AC ligament and includes no displacement on plain film radiography. A type I AC joint injury is treated with conservative management. Type II AC injury includes up to 50% displacement of the clavicle with an increase in the coracoclavicular distance on plain film radiography. Type III AC injury includes 50% to 100% displacement of the clavicle on plain film radiography.

27. **D.** The compression test involves putting pressure on the patient's carpal tunnel and holding the position for 60 seconds. This test is

positive when the patient's symptoms are reproduced with this maneuver. The compression test is the most sensitive test for carpal tunnel syndrome. Tinel's sign involves repetitively tapping over the median nerve as it passes through the carpal tunnel. This sign is positive when the tapping elicits the patient's symptoms. Tinel's sign is the most specific test for carpal tunnel syndrome. In Phalen's test, the patient holds both wrists in flexion against one another for 60 seconds. This test is positive when symptoms are reproduced. McMurray's test is used to identify a meniscal tear in the knee. Finkelstein's test is used to evaluate for de Quervain's tenosynovitis.

28. **C.** Provocative discogram with post-discogram CT evaluation is used to evaluate for discogenic back pain. This test involves injecting dye into the intervertebral disc via a percutaneous needle. When the pressure from the dye reproduces the patient's typical pain, the test is positive. On post-test CT evaluation, the dye is monitored for extravasation from the nucleus pulposus into the annulus fibrosus. There are five grades of potential fissuring in the annulus fibrosus. Grade 0 is no fissure. Grade I is a fissure that penetrates the inner third of the annulus. Grade II penetrates the middle third of the annulus. Grade III penetrates the outer third of the annulus. Grade IV penetrates circumferentially around the rim of the annulus. Patients with a positive provocative discography typically also have a grade III or greater annulus fissure.

29. **E.** All infants should be evaluated during the physical examination for evidence of developmental dysplasia of the hip (DDH). The Ortolani test is performed by flexing both hips to 90 degrees and then gently abducting them. If a palpable low-frequency "clunk" is appreciated, this is evidence of a congenitally dislocated hip. In the Barlow test, the femur is flexed and adducted with a posterior pressure applied. If the hip is unstable, the femur will be easily dislocated from the acetabulum and subsequently easily reduced. When DDH is suspected, ultrasonography is the test of choice. Some physicians advocate that ultrasonography should be used as a screening test for all infants regardless of physical examination. CT and/or MRI may be used for complicated cases.

30. **E.** The common peroneal nerve is a branch of the sciatic nerve. Injury to the common peroneal nerve will result in weakened dorsiflexion and foot eversion. An injury to the tibial nerve will result in impaired plantarflexion. Injury to the femoral nerve would result in impaired knee extension.

31. **E.** This patient most likely has plantar fasciitis. The diagnosis is made by history and physical examination. Conservative management is the first line of therapy and includes stretching, activity modification, and orthotics.

32. **D.** The Hawkins maneuver involves flexing the shoulder to 90 degrees in the plane of the scapula with the elbow in the flexed position. The shoulder is then moved firmly into internal rotation. If this maneuver

elicits pain, it is considered positive for an impingement. Another good test for impingement syndrome is to inject an anesthetic into the subacromial space. If the Hawkins maneuver is positive before the injection, but negative after the anesthetic has had a chance to work, then there is strong evidence for the diagnosis of impingement syndrome.

33. **A.** The typical patient with a supracondylar fracture is a child who reports having fallen onto an outstretched arm or other extension type of injury. In Gartland's classification, type I is nondisplaced. Type II is described by answer A. Type III has lost all cortex continuity.

34. **B.** The flexor retinaculum is a fibrous band of tissue that forms the six tunnels to the wrist. Each tunnel transmits extensor muscle tendons. In the first tunnel are the tendons of the abductor pollicis longus and extensor pollicis brevis muscles. The second tunnel contains the tendons of the extensor carpi radialis longus and extensor carpi radialis brevis muscles. The third tunnel contains the tendon of the extensor pollicis longus muscle. The fourth tunnel contains the tendons of the extensor digitorum and extensor indicis muscles. The fifth tunnel contains the tendon of the extensor digiti minimi. The sixth tunnel contains the tendon of the extensor carpi ulnaris muscle.

35. **C.** Patients with curvatures less than 20 degrees should be watched with serial examinations and radiographs, but not necessarily treated. Patients with curves between 20 and 40 degrees should be treated with full-time bracing. If the curve occurs at T8 or below, a plastic thoracolumbosacral orthosis (TLSO) may be used. If the curve is above the level of T8, a cervicothoracolumbosacral orthosis (CTLSO) or Milwaukee brace is indicated. Surgery is generally reserved for those patients with skeletal immaturity who have failed bracing treatment and have curves greater than 40 degrees, or in patients with curves greater than 50 degrees with functional impairment.

36. **E.** The quadriceps muscles are innervated by the femoral nerve and insert via the patellar ligament onto the patella. The function of the quadriceps is to primarily extend the knee. The rectus femoris arises from the anterior inferior iliac spine and crosses two joints. In addition to extending the knee, the rectus femoris also works to the flex the hip.

37. **E.** This patient most likely has slipped capital femoral epiphysis (SCFE). The patient will typically be an overweight male boy in puberty. The characteristic finding is for the patient to increase external rotation as the hip is flexed. Patients also typically have limited hip flexion, abduction, and internal rotation. Diagnosis should be confirmed with AP, lateral, and frog-leg radiographs. The "ice cream falling off the cone" sign on the radiograph is classic for SCFE.

38. **A.** This is Wilson's sign, and it is used to diagnose osteochondritis dissecans on the medial femoral condyle of the knee. As the knee is

extended to 30 degrees of flexion, the tibial spine abuts the medial femoral condyle. If an osteochondritis dissecans lesion is present on the medial femoral condyle, this will cause pain. When the knee is put into external rotation, pressure is taken off the lesion and the pain alleviates.

39. **D.** Schatzker types I, II, and III tibial plateau fractures involve only the lateral tibial plateau. Schatzker type V and VI fractures involve the medial and lateral portions of the tibial plateau. A type IV Schatzker tibial plateau fracture involves only the medial portion of the tibial plateau.

40. **C.** Club foot is a clinical diagnosis, and imaging studies are not necessary. Idiopathic cases of club foot may be treated with cast correction with or without Achilles tendon lengthening. Casting may be continued from birth until 6 months.

41. **D.** The diagnosis of interdigital neuroma is generally a clinical one. A common cause of an interdigital neuroma is tight-fitting shoes with narrow toe boxes that may compress the intermetatarsal ligament.

42. **E.** The typical patient with a Monteggia fracture is someone who reports falling onto an outstretched arm. Radiographs should be obtained. When a Monteggia fracture is confirmed, it should be staged. In the Bado staging system, type I (the most common type) involves an anterior radial head dislocation found along with an apex anterior proximal one-third ulna fracture. In a type II Bado Monteggia fracture, a posterior radial head dislocation is associated with an apex posterior proximal one-third ulna fracture. In a type III Bado Monteggia fracture, a lateral radial head dislocation is found with a proximal ulna metaphysical fracture. In a type IV Bado Monteggia fracture, an anterior radial head dislocation is found with a proximal one-third radius and ulna fracture. Types I, III, and IV are treated with open reduction and internal fixation followed by casting to 110 degrees of flexion. Type II fracture is treated with open reduction and internal fixation followed by casting in 70 degrees of flexion.

43. **A.** During the posterior approach to the hip, the large sciatic nerve is found exiting below the piriformis. The sciatic nerve is formed by the posterior divisions of the ventral rami of L5, S1, and S2. The sciatic nerve is the largest nerve in the body and divides halfway down the thigh into the common peroneal nerve and the tibial nerve.

44. **C.** The rotator cuff muscles consist of the supraspinatus, infraspinatus, teres minor, and subscapularis. The supraspinatus and infraspinatus muscles are innervated by the suprascapular nerve. The teres minor muscle is innervated by the axillary nerve. The subscapularis muscle is innervated by the upper and lower subscapular nerves.

45. **E.** The median nerve runs lateral to the brachial artery in the anterior elbow. Injury to the median nerve at this point may result in loss of

forearm pronation, wrist and digit flexion, thumb apposition, and loss of sensation in the lateral portion of the palm, including loss of sensation on the palmar surface of the first three digits.

46. **C.** This is Spurling's test. The maneuver described narrows the intervertebral foramen. In a patient with cervical radicular pain, cervical radiculopathy, or both, this maneuver may reproduce the patient's symptoms by applying additional stress to the involved nervous structures. Similarly, applying traction while flexing the head and rotating it to the opposite side relieves the pressure on the intervertebral foramen and should alleviate the symptoms. Patients with cervical spondylotic myelopathy may have a wide-based and/or unsteady gait and should be evaluated with plain films, CT, and MRI.

47. **D.** If pain is experienced in the AC joint, then AC joint disease is suspected. When a SLAP lesion is suspected, MRI is a helpful diagnostic tool. The gold standard for diagnosis of a SLAP lesion remains direct inspection and probing during arthroscopy.

48. **B.** Osteochondritis dissecans (OCD) is a condition in which a fragment of cartilage and subchondral bone separates from an intact articular surface. The fragment may completely or incompletely separate. OCD is generally thought to be a multifactorial disorder. In the elbow, for example, repetitive trauma and ischemia are thought to play a major role. In the ankle, particularly in the lateral malleolus, OCD is believed to be more related to trauma.

49. **D.** Thompson's test involves placing the patient in the prone position and passively flexing the knee. The Achilles is then squeezed. If the foot fails to go into plantarflexion, this is a positive Thompson's test and indicates an Achilles tendon rupture. This is not to be confused with Thomas's test, which is used to evaluate for hip flexor tightness. In Thomas's test, the patient lies in the supine position and flexes one hip, hugging it to the chest. If the opposite hip flexor is tight, the extended leg will raise off the table. If no hip flexor tightness is present, the extended leg will remain flat on the table.

50. **A.** In a total hip replacement, cement fixation offers the advantage of being the strongest fixation immediately after surgery. Patients with cement prostheses are weight-bearing as tolerated after surgery. With cementless procedures, patients must remain toe-touch weight-bearing (may put only about 10% of their weight onto the affected limb) for approximately 6 weeks after surgery. However, cementless procedures have the advantage of a stronger overall fixation once the bony ingrowth has occurred. In general, cemented procedures are preferred in elderly patients, and cementless procedures are preferred in younger patients.

Commonly Prescribed Medications (Adult Doses)

Acetaminophen (Tylenol) 650 mg PO q 4 hours as needed for pain (caution in hepatic failure or chronic alcohol use)

Acetaminophen/Codeine (Tylenol #2) 300/15 take 1–2 tab(s) PO q 4 hours as needed for mild to moderate pain (caution in hepatic failure or chronic alcohol use)

Acetaminophen/Codeine (Tylenol #3) 300/30 take 1–2 tab(s) PO q 4 hours as needed for mild to moderate pain (caution in hepatic failure or chronic alcohol use)

Acetaminophen/Codeine (Tylenol #4) 300/60 take 1–2 tab(s) PO q 4 hours as needed for mild to moderate pain (caution in hepatic failure or chronic alcohol use)

Acetaminophen/Hydrocodone (Vicodin) 500/5 take 1–2 tab(s) PO q 4 hours as needed for moderate to severe pain (caution in hepatic failure or chronic alcohol use)

Acetaminophen/Oxycodone (Percocet) 325/10 take 1–2 tab(s) PO q 4 hours as needed for moderate to severe pain

Acetaminophen/Propoxyphene napsylate (Darvocet) 325/50 take 1–2 tab(s) PO q 4 hours as needed for mild to moderate pain (caution in hepatic failure or chronic alcohol use)

Acetaminophen/Tramadol (Ultracet) 325/37.5 take 1–2 tab(s) PO q 4 hours as needed for pain (caution in hepatic failure or chronic alcohol use)

Aspirin 325 mg PO BID for thrombosis prophylaxis (take with food; caution with GI symptoms)

Aspirin/Hydrocodone (Lortab ASA) 500/5 take 1–2 tab(s) PO q 4 hours as needed for moderate to severe pain (take with food; caution with GI symptoms)

Aspirin/Oxycodone (Percodan) 325/4.5 take 1 tab PO q 6 hours as needed for moderate pain (take with food; caution with GI symptoms)

Calcium 1250 mg PO QD (take with food)

Enoxaparin (Lovenox) 30 mg SQ q 12 hours (or 40 mg SQ qd) for DVT prophylaxis (caution in renal failure)

Fentanyl transdermal (Duragesic) 25–100 mcg/hr patch q 72 hours

Heparin 5000 U SQ bid for DVT prophylaxis

Ibuprofen (Motrin) 100–800 mg PO q 6 hours as needed for pain (take with food; caution with doses above 300 TID; caution with GI symptoms)

Meloxicam (Mobic) 7.5–15 mg PO qd for pain (caution with GI symptoms, caution with renal disease)

Morphine (MS Contin) 15–30 mg PO q 8–12 hours for moderate to severe chronic pain

Morphine (MSIR) 15–30 mg PO q 4 hours for severe pain

Tramadol (Ultram) 50–100 mg PO q 4 hours as needed for moderate to severe pain

Warfarin (Coumadin) take as needed PO qd. Monitor PT/INR closely to keep INR within target range (often target INR = 2–3). Use for long-term anticoagulation.

D Glossary of Key Words, Terms, and Tests

Antalgic gait: Gait is marked by limping in order to avoid or reduce pain.

Anterior apprehension sign: Used to evaluate for anterior shoulder instability. The patient's arm is put into abduction, external rotation, and extension. A positive sign is elicited when the patient appears apprehensive with this maneuver. By the examiner placing posteriorly directed pressure to the anterior shoulder, stabilizing the humeral head in the glenoid fossa, the patient's apprehension should be alleviated.

Apley compression and distraction test: Used to evaluate for knee meniscus and ligament injury. The patient lies prone and the knee is flexed. The examiner puts the knee into internal and external rotation while applying a compression force. The examiner then applies a distraction force and continues to maneuver the knee into internal and external rotation. The test is positive for a meniscus injury if pain is elicited during compression but not distraction. Pain with compression *and* distraction is more likely to be a ligament injury and not a meniscus injury.

Arthrodesis: Immobilization, or fusion, of a joint

Atlas: C1 vertebra

Axis: C2 vertebra

Babinski reflex: Used to evaluate for an upper motor neuron lesion. A blunt instrument is scraped from the calcaneus of the patient along the lateral border of the foot to the first digit. If the patient extends the first digit and flexes the remaining digits, the patient has a Babinski reflex. The Babinski reflex should disappear at around 1 year of life in most people.

Bankart lesion: Tear of the anterior glenoid labrum

Barlow's test: Used to evaluate for developmental dysplasia of the hip (DDH) in an infant. The patient's femurs are flexed and adducted as the examiner applies a posteriorly directed pressure. The test is positive if the hips are easily dislocatable and reducible.

Cozen's test: Used to evaluate for lateral epicondylitis. The patient makes a fist, pronates the hand, and radially deviates the wrist against resistance. The test is positive when pain is elicited in the lateral epicondyle.

Fabere (or Patrick's) test: Used to evaluate for sacroiliac joint disease or hip disease. The patient lies supine and the patient's hip is flexed, abducted, and externally rotated into a figure-four position. The test is positive if pain is reproduced when inferiorly directed pressure is applied to the patient's flexed knee.

Finkelstein's test: Used to evaluate for de Quervain's tenosynovitis. The patient's thumb is passively adducted across the palm. The test is positive if pain is elicited.

Gerber lift-off test: Used to evaluate for subscapularis weakness. The patient's hand is placed behind the back with the palm facing posteriorly, and the patient pushes the hand off the back. If a lesion is present in the subscapularis, the patient will be unable to forcefully push off the spine.

Hill Sachs lesion: Compression fracture of the posterior humeral head

Hoffman's test: Used to evaluate for an upper motor neuron lesion. The patient's third proximal interphalangeal (PIP) joint is stabilized, and the distal interphalangeal (DIP) joint is flicked (briefly flexing it). If the patient's first interphalangeal joint or second DIP joint reflexively flexes, the test is positive for an upper motor neuron lesion.

Lachman's test: Used to evaluate for an anterior cruciate ligament (ACL) tear. The knee is flexed to 30 degrees and anteroposterior glide is assessed. A loose endpoint or excessive glide may reflect an ACL tear. This is the most sensitive physical examination test for an ACL tear.

McMurray's test: Used to evaluate for an injury of the posterior half of the medial meniscus. The patient lies supine and the knee is maximally flexed. The knee is put into external rotation, and a valgus stress is applied as the examiner slowly extends the patient's knee. A positive test is found if a palpable or audible click is appreciated in the joint line.

Neer test: Used to evaluate for shoulder impingement syndrome. The patient's shoulder is internally rotated and flexed in the scapular plane. The test is positive if pain is elicited.

O'Brien test: Used to evaluate for a superior labral anterior posterior (SLAP) or acromioclavicular (AC) injury. The patient's shoulder is flexed to 90 degrees, and the elbow is kept in full extension. The shoulder is put into 15 degrees of adduction, and the examiner applies an inferiorly directed force that the patient resists. The maneuver is repeated with the patient's hand in pronation. When pain is elicited in the shoulder with the hand in supination but not pronation, a SLAP lesion is suspected. If pain is elicited in the AC joint, an AC injury is suspected.

Ortolani test: Used to evaluate for DDH in an infant. The hips are flexed to 90 degrees and then gently abducted. The test is positive for a dislocated hip if there is a clunking sensation or sound with this maneuver.

Osteotomy: A surgery in which a bone, or piece of a bone, is removed

Phalen's test: Used to evaluate for carpal tunnel syndrome. The patient's hands are flexed and apposed for 60 seconds. The test is positive when symptoms are reproduced.

Radicular pain: Radiating, electric, bandlike pain caused by inflammation of a nerve root or compression of a dorsal root ganglion

Radiculopathy: Neurologic condition of loss that results in weakness, numbness, and/or diminished reflexes. It is caused by compression or ischemia of a nerve root.

Referred pain: Dull, aching, and difficult to localize pain. The pain is perceived in an area other than the site of pathology. This pathophysiology of referred pain is based on the principal of convergence, in which distinct areas of separate innervation share a similar pathway to the brain. The brain is unable to distinguish the original source of pain and so experiences the pain in multiple poorly defined areas.

Speed's test: Used to evaluate for bicipital tendonitis. The patient's forearm is supinated and arm flexion is resisted. The test is positive if pain is elicited.

Spondylolisthesis: Anterior or posterior slippage of one vertebrae in relation to the adjacent vertebra

Spondylolysis: A defect in the pars interarticularis

Spondylosis: Degenerative arthritis of the spine

Spurling's test: Used to evaluate for radicular symptoms. The patient's head is put into extension, lateral flexion, and gentle compression. A positive test is found when the patient experiences reproduction of symptoms.

Subluxation: This term refers to an incomplete or partial dislocation.

Trendelenburg gait: Used to evaluate for a weak gluteus medius. The patient's hip will slide inferiorly toward the side of the lesion in a Trendelenburg gait.

Wilson's sign: Used to evaluate for medial femoral condyle OCD. The patient's knee is flexed to 90 degrees and internally rotated. In internal rotation, the knee is slowly extended. The test is positive if pain is elicited at about 30 degrees of extension. External rotation of the knee should alleviate the pain.

Yergason's test: Used to evaluate for bicipital tendonitis and bicipital instability. The patient's elbow is flexed to 90 degrees, and the patient supinates the forearm against resistance. The test is positive if pain is elicited.

Yocum test: Used to evaluate for supraspinatus tendonitis. The patient's shoulder is flexed to 90 degrees, and the patient's arm is flexed to 60 degrees. The shoulder is then put into firm internal rotation. The test is positive if pain is elicited.

Zygapophyseal joints: Synovial joints articulating between the inferior articular processes of one vertebra and the superior articular processes of the adjacent inferior vertebra

Suggested Additional Reading

CHAPTER 1

Bogduk N. The anatomy and pathophysiology of neck pain. *Physical Medicine & Rehabilitation Clinics of North America* 2003; 14(3): 455–72.

Koivikko MP, Myllynen P, Santavirta S. Fracture dislocations of the cervical spine: a review of 106 conservatively and operatively treated patients. *European Spine Journal* 2004; 13(7): 610–6.

Maeda T, Saito T, Harimaya K, et al. Atlantoaxial instability in neck retraction and protrusion positions in patients with rheumatoid arthritis. *Spine* 2004; 29(7): 757–62.

Rathmell JP, Aprill C, Bogduk N. Cervical transforaminal injection of steroids. *Anesthesiology* 2004; 100(6): 1595–600.

Reindl R, Sen M, Aebi M. Anterior instrumentation for traumatic C1-2 instability. *Spine* 2003; 28(17): E329–33.

CHAPTER 2

Mothadi NG, Vellet AD, Clark ML, et al. A prospective, double-blind comparison of magnetic resonance imaging and arthroscopy in the evaluation of patients presenting with shoulder pain. *Journal of Shoulder & Elbow Surgery* 2004; 13(3): 258–65.

Quillen DM, Wuchner M, Hatch RL. Acute shoulder injuries. *American Family Physician* 2004; 70(10): 1947–54.

Rahme H, Mattsson P, Larsson S. Stability of cemented all-polyethylene keeled glenoid components. A radiostereometric study with a two-year follow-up. *Journal of Bone & Joint Surgery* (Br) 2004; 86(6): 856–60.

Sperling JW, Cofield RH, Schleck C. Rotator cuff repair in patients fifty years of age and younger. *Journal of Bone and Joint Surgery* (Am) 2004; 86-A(10): 2212–5.

CHAPTER 3

Dunkow PD, Jatti M, Muddu BN. A comparison of open and percutaneous techniques in the surgical treatment of tennis elbow. *Journal of Bone & Joint Surgery* (Br) 2004; 86(5): 701–4.

Pavelka M, Rhomberg M, Estermann D, et al. Decompression without anterior transposition: an effective minimally invasive technique for cubital tunnel syndrome. *Minimally Invasive Neurosurgery* 2004; 47(2): 119–23.

Trinh KV, Phillips SD, Ho E, Damsma K. Acupuncture for the alleviation of lateral epicondyle pain: a systematic review. *Rheumatology* 2004; 43(9): 1085–90.

Wada T, Isogai S, Ishii S, Yamashita T. Debridement arthroplasty for primary osteoarthritis of the elbow. *Journal of Bone & Joint Surgery* (Am) 2004; 86-A(2): 233–41.

Williams RJ 3rd, Urgquart ER, Altchek DW. Medial collateral ligament tears in the throwing athlete. *Instructional Course Lectures* 2004; 53: 579–86.

CHAPTER 4

Armstrong T, Devor W, Borschel L, Contreras R. Intracarpal steroid injection is safe and effective for short-term management of carpal tunnel syndrome. *Muscle & Nerve* 2004; 29(1): 82–8.

Handoll HH, Vaghela MV. Interventions for treating mallet finger injuries. *Cochrane Database of Systematic Reviews* 2004; (3): CD004574.

MacDermid JC, Wessel J. Clinical diagnosis of carpal tunnel syndrome: a systematic review. *Journal of Hand Therapy* 2004; 17(2): 309–19.

Matsuzaki H, Yoshizu T, Tsubokawa N, et al. Long-term clinical and neurologic recovery in the hand after surgery for severe cubital tunnel syndrome. *Journal of Hand Surgery* (Am) 2004; 29(3): 373–8.

Meenagh GK, Patton J, Kynes C, Wrigth GD. A randomised controlled trial of intra-articular corticosteroid injection of the carpometacarpal joint of the thumb in osteoarthritis. *Annals of the Rheumatic Diseases* 2004; 63(10): 1260–3.

Senall JA, Failla JM, Bouffard JA, van Holsbeeck M. Ultrasound for the early diagnosis of clinically suspected scaphoid fracture. *Journal of Hand Surgery* (Am) 2004; 29(3): 400–5.

CHAPTER 5

Bono CM, Lee CK. Critical analysis of trends in fusion for degenerative disc disease over the past 20 years: influence of technique on fusion rate and clinical outcome. *Spine* 2004; 29(4): 455–63.

Mummaneni PV, Haid RW, Rodts GE. Lumbar interbody fusion: state-of-the-art technical advances. Invited submission from the Joint Section Meeting on Disorders of the Spine and Peripheral Nerves, March 2004. *Journal of Neurosurgery* 2004; 1(1): 24–30.

Pauza KJ, Howell S, Dreyfuss P, et al. A randomized, placebo-controlled trial of intradiscal electrothermal therapy for the treatment of discogenic low back pain. *Spine Journal* 2004; 4(1): 27–35.

Rao RD, Singrakhia MD. Painful osteoporotic vertebral fracture. Pathogenesis, evaluation, and roles of vertebroplasty and kyphoplasty in its management. *Journal of Bone & Joint Surgery* (Am) 2003; 85-A(10): 2010–22.

Shufflebarger HL, Geck MJ, Clark CE. The posterior approach for lumbar and thoracolumbar adolescent idiopathic scoliosis: posterior shortening and pedicle screws. *Spine* 2004; 29(3): 269–76.

Vad VB, Bhat AL, Lutz GE, Cammisa F. Transforaminal epidural steroid injections in lumbosacral radiculopathy: a prospective randomized study. *Spine* 2002; 27(1): 11–16.

Van Kleef M, Weber WE, Kessels A, et al. Efficacy and validity of radiofrequency neurotomy for chronic lumbar zygapophyseal joint pain. *Spine* 2000; 25: 1270–7.

CHAPTER 6

Aderinto J, Brenkel IJ. Pre-operative predictors of the requirement for blood transfusion following total hip replacement. *Journal of Bone & Joint Surgery* (Br) 2004; 86(7): 970–3.

Chung WK, Liu D, Foo LS. Mini-incision total hip replacement—surgical technique and early results. *Journal of Orthopedic Surgery* 2004; 12(1): 19–24.

Jolles BM, Bogoch ER. Surgical approach for total hip arthroplasty: direct lateral or posterior? *Journal of Rheumatology* 2004; 31(9): 1790–6.

Kocher MS, Bishop JA, Hresko MT, et al. Prophylactic pinning of the contralateral hip after unilateral slipped capital femoral epiphysis. *Journal of Bone & Joint Surgery* (Am) 2004; 86-A(12): 2658–65.

Kwong LM. Hip fracture and venous thromboembolism in the elderly. *Journal of Orthopedic Advances* 2004; 13(3):139–48.

Margo K, Drezner J, Motzkin D. Evaluation and management of hip pain: an algorithmic approach. *Journal of Family Practice* 2003; 52(8): 607–17.

Sikand M, Wenn R, Moran CG. Mortality following surgery for undisplaced intracapsular hip fractures. *Injury* 2004; 35(10): 1015–9.

Upadhyay A, Jain P, Mishra P, et al. Delayed internal fixation of fractures of the neck of the femur in young adults. A prospective, randomized study comparing closed and open reduction. *Journal of Bone & Joint Surgery* (Br) 2004; 86(7): 1035–40.

CHAPTER 7

Aglietti P, Giron F, Buzzi R, et al. Anterior cruciate ligament reconstruction: bone-patellar tendon-bone compared with double semitendinosus and gracilis tendon grafts. A prospective, randomized clinical trial. *Journal of Bone & Joint Surgery* (Am) 2004, 86-A(10): 2143–55.

Elkus M, Ranawat CS, Rasquinha VJ, et al. Total knee arthroplasty for severe valgus deformity. Five- to fourteen-year follow-up. *Journal of Bone & Joint Surgery* (Am) 2004; 86-A(12): 2671–6.

Heintjes E, Berger MY, Bierma-Zeinstra SM, et al. Pharmacotheraphy for patellofemoral pain syndrome. *Cochrane Database of Systematic Reviews* 2004; 3:CD003470.

Lohmander LS, Ostenberg A, Englund M, Roos H. High prevalence of knee osteoarthritis, pain, and functional limitations in female soccer players twelve years after anterior cruciate ligament injury. *Arthritis & Rheumatism* 2004; 50(10): 3145–52.

Smirk C, Morris H. The anatomy and reconstruction of the medial patellofemoral ligament. *Knee* 2003; 10(3): 221–7.

Wright RW, McLean M, Matava MJ, Shively RA. Osteochondritis dissecans of the knee: long-term results of excision of the fragment. *Clinical Orthopedics & Related Research* 2004; 424: 239–43.

CHAPTER 8

Anderson T, Montgomery F, Carlsson A. Uncemented STAR total ankle prostheses. *Journal of Bone & Joint Surgery* (Am) 2004; 86-A Suppl 1(Pt 2): 103–11.

Chen CY, Huang PJ, Kao KF, et al. Surgical reconstruction for chronic lateral instability of the ankle. *Injury* 2004; 35(8): 809–13.

Ebell MH. Evaluating the patient with an ankle or foot injury. *American Family Physician* 2004; 70(8): 1535–6.

Jennings AG, Sefton GK, Newman RJ. Repair of acute rupture of the Achilles tendon: a new technique using polyester tape without external splintage. *Annals of the Royal College of Surgeons of England* 2004; 86(6): 445–8.

McBryde AM Jr., Hoffman JL. Injuries to the foot and ankle in athletes. *Southern Medical Journal* 2004; 97(8): 738–41.

Schmidt R, Cordier E, Bertsch C, et al. Reconstruction of the lateral ligaments: do the anatomical procedures restore physiologic ankle kinematics? *Foot and Ankle International* 2004; 25(1): 31–36.

Wasserman LR, Saltzman CL, Amendola A. Minimally invasive ankle reconstruction: current scope and indications. *Orthopedics Clinics of North America* 2004; 35(2): 247–53.

Index

Note: Page numbers with an *f* indicate figures; those with a *t* indicate tables; those with a *b* indicate boxes.

Acetaminophen, 153
Achilles tendon injuries, 117–118, 152
ACL. *See* Anterior cruciate ligament injury
Acromioclavicular (AC) joint injuries, 26–27, 26*t*
Acromions, 21, 22*t*
Adhesive capsulitis, 18–19
Adolescents. *See also* Children
  Legg-Calvé-Perthes disease in, 108
  SCFE in, 81–83
  scoliosis in, 57–58
Ankle, 113–129. *See also* Foot
  Achilles tendon injuries of, 117–118
  anatomy of, 113–114
  bony impingement in, 119–120
  calcaneal fracture of, 127
  ligaments of, 115*f*
  osteochondritis dissecans of, 118–119
  Ottawa rules for, 116, 117*b*
  pain in, 120–121
  sprain of, 114–117, 115*f*, 115*t*, 116*f*, 117*b*, 147
  talus fracture of, 127–129, 128*f*, 129*t*
  tibial fracture and, 123–126, 124*f*–126*f*, 125*t*
Annuloplasty, 61
Annulus fibrosus fissure, 60, 61*t*, 149
Anterior bony impingement, 119–120

Anterior cervical discectomy and fusion (ACDF)
  for radiculopathy, 6
  for spondylotic myelopathy, 7
Anterior cruciate ligament (ACL) injury, 97–99, 98*f*
Anterior drawer test, 115–116, 116*f*
Apley test, 103, 104*f*, 146
Apprehension test, 16*f*
Arthritis
  atlantoaxial subluxation with, 11
  carpal tunnel syndrome and, 44
  of hand, 49–50, 50*f*
  of hip, 82–87, 84*f*
  of knee, 85, 105–108, 106*f*
  septic, 83
  Z-joint disease with, 8
Arthrodesis
  atlantoaxial, 12*t*
  odontoid, 12
Arthrosis, wrist, 52
Atlantoaxial rotary subluxation, 11, 12*t*
Atlanto-occipital dislocation, 9–10
Autogenous osteochondral grafting, 85
Autologous chondrocyte implantation (ACI), 85
Avascular necrosis (AVN)
  of femur, 77, 82, 89, 90, 93
  of lunate bone, 52, 147
  osteoarthritis and, 83
  of scaphoid bone, 54
  of talus, 129

Axis
 fracture of, 10–11
 neck pain from, 6–8
 spondylolisthesis of, 8–9, 9t

Babinski's sign, 4, 7
Bado classification, 40t, 151
Bankart lesion, 15, 17
Barlow's test, 75
Biceps muscle, 4t
 anatomy of, 13–14
 disorders of, 23–25, 24f
 SLAP lesion of, 23–25, 24f, 152
 tendonitis of, 23–25, 24f
Bigliani classification, 21, 22t
Brachial plexus, 14, 28, 31
"Bucket-handle" lesion, 102

Calcaneal fracture, 127
Capsulitis, adhesive, 18–19
Carpal tunnel syndrome, 43–46
 compression test for, 24–25,
  148–149
 Phalen's test for, 45, 46f, 149
 Tinel's sign in, 44, 45f, 149
Caterall staging of LCPD, 78t
Cervical spine, 1–12
 anatomy of, 1–3, 148
 functions of, 1
 radiculopathy of, 3–6, 4f, 4t
 spondylosis of, 8
 spondylotic myelopathy of, 6–7
 Z-joint disease of, 7–8, 144
Cheliectomy, 123
Children. See also Adolescents
 clavicular fracture in, 28
 club foot in, 114, 151
 DDH in, 74–77
 hip synovitis in, 79–81
Chondroitin sulfate, 85
Chondromalacia, 108
Clavicular fracture, 27–28
Club foot, 114, 151
Cobb angle, 57
Codeine, 153
Colles' fracture, 52–53, 53f
Compression test, 24–25, 148–149
Continuous passive motion
 (CPM) machines, 108

Coracobrachialis muscle, 13–14
Cozen's test, 32
Cubital tunnel syndrome,
 35–36, 145

DDH (developmental dysplasia
 of the hip), 74–77, 149
Deep vein thrombosis (DVT)
 after hip fracture, 92–93
 after hip replacement, 86
 from knee replacement, 108
Deltoid muscle, 13
De Quervain's tenosynovitis,
 46–48, 47f, 147
Dermatomes
 cervical, 4f
 lumbar, 63f–66f, 68t
 sacral, 67f, 68f
 thoracic, 4f
Developmental dysplasia of the
 hip (DDH), 74–77, 149
"Dinner fork" deformity, 52–53, 53f
Discogram, 149
Dislocation
 atlanto-occipital, 9–10
 hip, 87–89
Down syndrome, 11
Drawer test, 115–116, 116f
DVT. See Deep vein thrombosis
Dysdiadochokinesis, 6
Dysplastic spondylolisthesis,
 68–69, 70f

Elbow, 30–41
 anatomy of, 30–31, 151–152
 cubital tunnel syndrome of,
  35–36
 epicondylitis of, 31–33
 golfer's, 31–33
 humeral fracture near, 36–37
 Monteggia fracture of, 40–41,
  40f, 151
 osteochondritis dissecans of,
  34–35, 152
 radial head fracture of, 39
 supracondylar fracture of,
  37–39, 38f
 tennis, 31–33
 ulnar ligament injury of, 33–34

Enoxaparin, 154
Epicondylitis, 31–33, 144
Equinovarus deformity, 114, 151

Fabere's test, 59, 60*f*
Fasciitis, plantar, 120–121, 149
Fentanyl, 154
Finkelstein's test, 47*f*, 147
Foot, 113–129. *See also* Ankle
    club, 114
    hallux rigidus of, 122–123
    hallux valgus of, 121–122, 121*f*
    interdigital neuroma of,
        123, 151
    plantar fasciitis of,
        120–121, 149
Forearm, 30–41. *See also* Elbow
Fracture
    axis, 10–11
    calcaneal, 127
    clavicular, 27–28
    Colles', 52–53, 53*f*
    hip, 89–93, 90*f*, 91*t*
    humeral, 28–29, 36–37
    intertrochanteric, 90*f*, 91*f*, 92*t*
    Monteggia, 40–41, 40*f*, 151
    odontoid, 11–12
    osteoporotic, 70–72
    patella, 110–111
    radial, 39, 52–53, 53*f*, 54*f*
    scaphoid, 53–55, 55*f*, 148
    supracondylar, 37–39, 38*f*
    talus, 127–129, 128*f*, 129*t*
    tibial, 123–126, 124*f*–126*f*,
        125*t*
    tibial plateau, 111–112
    vertebral compression, 70–72
Frozen shoulder, 18–19

Gait, Trendelenburg, 65, 68*t*,
    77, 145
Ganglion, wrist, 50–51
Garden classification of hip
    fractures, 90, 91*t*, 146
Gartland classification, 37,
    38*t*, 150
Gerber's lift-off test, 21, 24
Glenoid osteotomy, 17–18
Glucosamine sulfate, 85

Golfer's elbow, 31–33
Gout, 83

Hallux rigidus, 122–123
Hallux valgus, 121–122, 121*f*
hamstrings, 94
Hand, 42–55. *See also* Wrist
Hawkins classification, 128–129,
    129*t*
Hawkins' test, 20–21, 20*f*,
    149–150
hemochromatosis, 83
Hemophilia, 83
Heparin. *See* Warfarin
Hill-Sachs lesion, 15, 17
Hip, 73–93
    anatomy of, 73–74
    developmental dysplasia of,
        74–77, 149
    dislocation of, 87–89
    fracture of, 89–93, 90*f*, 91*f*,
        91*t*, 92*t*, 146
    Legg-Calvé-Perthes disease of,
        77–79, 78*f*
    osteoarthritis of, 83–86, 84*f*
    pain in, 79–81
    replacement of, 85–87
    rheumatoid arthritis of, 86–87
    slipped capital femoral
        epiphysis of, 81–83, 108,
        109, 145, 150
    transient synovitis of, 79–81
Hoffman's sign, 4, 6–7
Humeral fracture
    distal, 36–37
    proximal, 28–29
    supracondylar, 37–39, 38*f*
Hydrocodone, 153
Hyperlordosis, 77

Ibuprofen, 154
IDET (intradiscal electrothermal)
    annuloplasty, 61
Iliopsoas muscle, 73
Impingement syndrome
    of ankle, 119–120
    of shoulder, 19–23, 20*f*, 22*f*,
        146, 150
Infraspinatus muscle, 15, 21, 151

Interdigital neuroma, 123, 151
Intertrochanteric fracture, 90f, 91f, 92t
Intradiscal electrothermal (IDET) annuloplasty, 61
Isthmic spondylolisthesis, 68–69, 70f

Kienbock's disease, 52, 147
Knee, 94–112
    anatomy of, 94–95, 150
    anterior cruciate ligament injury of, 97–99, 98f
    medial collateral ligament injury of, 99–101, 100f, 146
    meniscus injuries of, 102–105, 104f, 105f
    Osgood-Schlatter disease of, 95–96
    osteoarthritis of, 85, 105–108, 106f
    osteochondritis dissecans of, 96–97, 146, 150–152
    pain in, 83, 108–111, 109f
    patellofemoral disorders of, 108–111, 109f, 146, 148
    posterior cruciate ligament injury of, 101–102
    replacement of, 107–108
    tibial plateau fracture of, 111–112
Kyphoplasty, 71–72, 144–145

LBP. See Low back pain
Legg-Calvé-Perthes disease (LCPD), 77–79, 78f
    knee pain from, 108, 109
    osteoarthritis and, 83
    staging of, 78t
Lhermitte's sign, 6
Low back pain (LBP), 58–62, 145
    annulus fibrosus fissure with, 60, 61t, 149
    chronic, 58, 61, 147
    hip dysplasia with, 77
    Patrick's test for, 59, 60f
Lumbar spine. See Thoracolumbar spine

Lumbosacral radiculopathy, 62–68, 63f–67f, 68t, 145
Lunate bone necrosis, 52, 147

MCL. See Medial collateral ligament injury
McMurray's test, 103–104, 105f, 146–147
Medial collateral ligament (MCL) injury, 99–101, 100f, 146
Meloxicam, 154
Meniscus injuries, 102–105, 104f, 105f
Milwaukee brace, 58, 150
Monteggia fracture, 40–41, 40f, 40t, 151
Morphine, 154
Mosaicplasty, 85
Myelopathy, spondylotic, 6–7

Neck. See Cervical spine
Neer's test, 20–21, 146
Neuroma, interdigital, 123, 151
Nonsteroidal anti-inflammatory drugs (NSAIDs), 153–154

O'Brien's compression test, 24–25, 148–149
OCD. See Osteochondritis dissecans
Odontoid fracture, 11–12
Orthotics, 58, 122–123, 150
Ortolani's test, 75, 149
Osgood-Schlatter disease, 95–96, 146
Osteoarthritis (OA). See also Rheumatoid arthritis
    of hip, 77, 83–86, 84f
    of knee, 85, 105–108, 106f
    from SCFE, 82–83
    with Z-joint disease, 8
Osteochondritis dissecans (OCD)
    of ankle, 118–119
    of elbow, 34–35, 152
    of knee, 96–97, 146, 150–152
Osteochondrodysplasia, 114, 151
Osteoporosis, 70–72, 144–145

Osteosynthesis, 12
Osteotomy, glenoid, 17–18
Ottawa ankle rules, 116, 117b
Oxycodone, 153

Paget's disease, 83
Patella fracture, 110–111
Patellofemoral disorders,
    108–110, 109f, 146, 148
Patrick's test, 59, 60f
Pavlik harness, 76, 77
PCL. See Posterior cruciate
    ligament injury
Pectoralis muscles, 13, 14
Phalen's test, 45, 46f, 149
Pitching injuries, 33–34
Plantar fasciitis, 120–121, 149
Platysma muscle, 1–2, 148
Polymethylmethacrylate
    (PMMA), 71, 145
Posterior cruciate ligament (PCL)
    injury, 101–102
Propoxyphene napsylate, 153
Pulmonary embolism (PE), 86,
    92–93

Q-angle, 108–109, 109f, 146
Quadriceps, 74, 94, 150
Quervain's tenosynovitis, 46–48,
    47f, 147

Radial fracture, 39t, 52–53, 53f,
    54f
Radiculopathy
    cervical, 3–6, 4f, 4t
    lumbosacral, 62–68, 63f–67f,
        68t, 145
Research projects, 130–131
Residency programs, 130
Review questions, 132–143
Rheumatoid arthritis (RA).
    See also Osteoarthritis
    atlantoaxial subluxation with, 11
    carpal tunnel syndrome and, 44
    of hand, 49–50, 50f
    of hip, 86–87
Rotator cuff, 19–23, 20f, 22f, 144
    muscles of, 14
    tendonitis of, 25–26

Sacroiliac joint pain, 58, 60–61
Salter-Harris classification,
    124–125, 125t, 147
Salter-Thomson classification, 78t
Scaphoid fracture, 53–55,
    55f, 148
SCFE. See Slipped capital
    femoral epiphysis
Schatzker classification, 111, 151
Sciatic nerve injury, 89
Scoliosis, 57–58
Shoulder, 13–29
    acromioclavicular joint injuries
        of, 26–27, 26t
    anatomy of, 13–15, 14f,
        148, 151
    biceps disorders, 23–25, 24f
    capsulitis of, 18–19
    clavicular fracture of, 27–28
    frozen, 18–19
    humeral fracture of, 28–29
    impingement syndrome of,
        19–23, 20f, 22f, 146, 150
    instability of, 15–18, 16f
    rotator cuff disease of, 19–23,
        20f, 22f
    rotator cuff tendonitis, 25–26
SLAP lesion. See Superior labral
    anterior posterior lesion
Slipped capital femoral epiphysis
    (SCFE), 81–83, 145, 150
    knee pain from, 108, 109
Speed test, 24, 146
Spina bifida, 114
Splenius muscles, 2–3
Spondylolisthesis, 8–9, 9t,
    68–69, 70f
Spondylosis, cervical, 8
Spondylotic myelopathy, 6–7
Spurling's test, 3–4, 5f, 8, 152
Stenosing tenosynovitis, 48–49
Sternocleidomastoid muscle, 1
Subcapularis tear, 21
Subluxation
    atlantoaxial, 11, 12t
    bicipital, 24
Superior labral anterior posterior
    (SLAP) lesion, 23–25,
    24f, 152

Supracondylar fracture, 37–39, 38*f*
Supraspinatus muscle, 14–15, 151
Synovitis, hip, 79–81

Talus fracture, 127–129, 128*f*, 129*t*
Tendonitis
  Achilles, 117–118
  bicipital, 23–25, 24*f*
  rotator cuff, 25–26, 144
Tennis elbow, 31–33
Tenosynovitis
  de Quervain's, 46–48, 47*f*, 147
  stenosing, 48–49
Teres minor muscle, 15, 21
Thomas's test, 152
Thompson's test, 118, 152
Thoracolumbar spine, 56–72
  anatomy of, 56–57
  low back pain and, 58–62, 60*f*, 61*t*
  osteoporotic fracture of, 70–72
  radiculopathy of, 62–68, 63*f*–67*f*, 68*t*
  scoliosis, 57–58
  spondylolisthesis of, 68–69, 70*f*
Tibial fracture, 123–126, 124*f*–126*f*, 125*t*
Tibial plateau fracture, 111–112
Tinel's sign, 35–36, 149
Total hip replacement (THR), 85–87, 152
Total knee replacement (TKR), 94, 107–108
Tramadol, 153–154
Transient synovitis (TS), 79–81

Trapezius muscle, 2
Trendelenburg gait, 65, 68t, 77, 145
Trethowan's sign, 82
Triceps muscle, 31
Trigger finger, 48–49

Vertebroplasty, 71–72

Wartenberg's sign, 36, 145
Warfarin, 86, 108, 154
Wilson's disease, 83
Wilson's test, 96, 147, 150–151
Wrist, 42–55
  anatomy of, 42–43
  arthritis of, 49–50
  arthrosis of, 52
  carpal tunnel syndrome of, 43–46, 45*f*, 46*f*
  Colles' fracture of, 52–53, 53*f*, 54*f*
  de Quervain's tenosynovitis of, 46–48, 47*f*
  ganglion of, 50–51
  Kienbock's disease of, 52
  scaphoid fracture of, 53–55, 55*f*
  stenosing tenosynovitis of, 48–49

Yersagon's test, 24*f*

Zygapophyseal joints, 3, 56
  disease of, 7–8, 61, 144
  pain from, 58–60
  radiculopathy from, 62
  spondylolisthesis of, 9*t*

Additional Praise for Blueprints *Orthopedics*

"Blueprints *Orthopedics* seems to cover just the right amount of info needed as a med student."

—1st year resident, Orthopaedic Surgery, Temple University

"The Q&A section is great. There is a paucity of Q&A out there for orthopaedics review for med students. Going into orthopaedics, my friends and I often lamented not having the same kind of review at our fingertips that our friends going into internal medicine or pediatrics had. Also, I think the book's organization is well put together anatomically, allowing for ease in reading and consultation."

—1st year Orthopedics Resident, University Hospitals of Cleveland/
Case Western Reserve University

"Blueprints *Orthopedics* provides a good source of basic orthopaedic knowledge in each of the orthopaedic subspecialties that will give a 3rd or 4th year medical student a good foundation for any orthopaedic rotation. Strengths include the explanation of surgical anatomy, helping students prepare for possible pimping questions during OR time; the emphasis on common surgical procedures, helping students become aware of what procedures they are most likely to encounter during a rotation; and the inclusion of risk factors/differential diagnoses, so students may be able to educate patients as to what they should avoid or expect in the course of disease."

—4th year medical student, Albany Medical College

"Blueprints *Orthopedics* is a very good book. It offers a concise presentation of material that can be read quickly and be reread if refreshment is needed. The physical exam sections are very high yield. Few other resources cover this material in a manageable fashion for med students. Really there is no other book available now that covers this information in a concise manner at a reasonable price."

—1st year Orthopedics Resident, Southern Illinois University

"The length is a definite advantage of this book. It is short enough to read the weekend before your elective and to give you an overview of what is to come. Most textbooks overestimate the amount of free time that medical students have to spend reading long-winded authors; however, this book does not. The organization of this book is very clear and the language is very accessible. It is anatomically sorted and medical terms/signs are overall well defined. The high yield anatomy sections introducing the chapters provide a helpful anatomical guide without belaboring clinically useless details. These high-quality, well written anatomical reviews are the kind that most students sadly do not routinely receive in medical school, emphasizing only the important details that affect diagnosis and treatment. The cost makes the book very reasonably priced considering the prices of comparable hardcover textbooks."

—3rd year medical student, UMDNJ/New Jersey Medical School